More Praise for
You Are Not Your Illness

"*You Are Not Your Illness* offers us a way to live successfully with a life-threatening illness or disability, helping us to see that we can choose to experience inner peace and healing regardless of the state of our body. It is a book of strength and hope that offers guidance for all of us ... written by a courageous woman who herself has multiple sclerosis and knows of what she speaks."
—Gerald G. Jampolsky, M.D., author of *Love Is Letting Go of Fear*

"An inspiring story of courage and sound principles for living in harmony with a life-threatening illness."
—Robert F. Lehman, President, The Fetzer Institute

"It is difficult to decide which one admires most—the author's courage or her wisdom. [*You Are Not Your Illness*] has important messages for everyone, for we all have a debilitating, life-threatening disease, the one called aging. What the author learned painfully, through the tragic, steady enfeebling of multiple sclerosis, we all have to learn. The book makes a most powerful point, namely that real healing has little to do with our state of physical health. The reader's response ... is likely to be profound gratitude for Linda's generous gift."
—Willis Harman, President, Institute of Noetic Sciences

"It takes an immense amount of courage to live with a serious illness —and that much more to turn it into a victory for the Soul. This inspiring book is about such a victory. It will touch your heart and show you a blueprint for finding meaning in life's challenges."
—H. Ronald Hulnick, Ph.D.,
President, University of Santa Monica
A Center for the Study and Practice of Spiritual Psychology

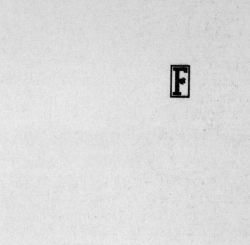

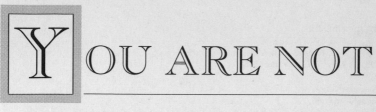

YOU ARE NOT
YOUR ILLNESS

Seven Principles for
Meeting the Challenge

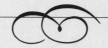

Linda Noble Topf, M.A.

with

Hal Zina Bennett, Ph.D.

A FIRESIDE BOOK

Published by Simon & Schuster

New York   London   Toronto   Sydney   Tokyo   Singapore

FIRESIDE
Rockefeller Center
1230 Avenue of the Americas
New York, New York 10020

Designed by Richard Oriolo

Manufactured in the United States of America

10 9 8 7 6 5 4

Library of Congress Cataloging-in-Publication Data

Topf, Linda Noble.
    You are not your illness : seven principles for meeting
the challenge / Linda Noble Topf with Hal Zina Bennett.
        p.   cm.
    "A Fireside book."
    Includes bibliographical references.
    1. Medicine and psychology.   2. Chronic diseases—
Psychological aspects.   3. Multiple
sclerosis—Psychological aspects.
I. Bennett, Hal Zina.   II. Title.
R726.5.T658   1995
155.9'16—dc20   94-39618
                                                       CIP

ISBN 0-684-80124-8

Grateful acknowledgment is given to the following for permission to reprint copyrighted material that
appears in this work.

Excerpts from *Future of Man* and other quotes by P. Teilhard de Chardin. Copyright Editions du
Seuil. Reprinted by permission.

From *How to Survive the Loss of a Love* by Melba Colgrove, Ph.D., Harold Bloomfield, M.D., and Peter
McWilliams, published by Prelude Press, 8159 Santa Monica Boulevard, Los Angeles, California
90046, 1-800-LIFE-101.

From *Getting the Love You Want* by Harville Hendrix, published by HarperCollins Publishers, Incorporated. Copyright 1988. Reprinted by permission of the author.

From *Illness as Metaphor* by Susan Sontag, published by Farrar, Straus & Giroux. Copyright 1977,
1978. Reprinted by permission.

continued on page 254

To Matt = 18/3/99

This book is dedicated to
each of us who travels further than
the obstacles put before us.
Thus, we will know a different quality of loving.

*May God Bless you
on your journey home.
Peace,*

Sinada

Nothing is precious except that part of you which is in other people and that part of others which is in you. Up there, on high, everything is one.

Pierre Teilhard de Chardin

Contents

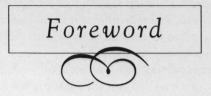

Foreword

Y ou Are Not Your Illness is about something that should matter to all of us. It is about life and love and healing. If I had the power, I would have everyone read it. Why would I do that? Because Linda has learned the lessons we all need to be aware of.

I receive many manuscripts from enlightened people. What enlightens them? AIDS, cancer, multiple sclerosis, and accidental deaths of loved ones. But why wait for enlightenment to come in this way? Why not read this book and learn these lessons ahead of time? Then you will be able to live a full life prepared for the difficulties we all meet.

I am fond of asking audiences if life is fair. The majority always answers, NO! I disagree; life is fair. We all have our difficulties. We need to learn how to deal with them. If there hasn't been someone in your life to help you learn how to work with difficulties, then let Linda's book guide you.

You Are Not Your Illness can show you who you are. It can help you hold up the mirror so you can see your true self and your beauty. This is not about perfection but about achieving completeness in your life and healing.

You will be asked to look at your conception of what health is. You will learn how to be healthy despite your physical afflictions.

You will learn to find the passion that can be the energy that leads you to discover a new life. This does not mean you will not feel the anger and grief and all the other emotions that are normal in times of crisis and despair.

However, what you will see is what happens to you and the "Beast" when kissed by "Beauty." You are the Beauty who can change everything in your life. No one else can do it for you. This book can only help you find what is in you. You must realize that the strength and the inspiration are inside you. Let this book help you raise the lid and release both.

We are all wounded, but we are not all victims. If you learn how to use your inner strength and your spiritual resources, you will always have choices and be empowered to make changes or find inner peace.

I feel there are two main themes to a healed life. One is finding a path in life, a way of contributing love to the world. This is not found by being intellectual and logical; that leads to your becoming path-o-logical. It is found by exploring your inner darkness, your feelings and your happiness. Linda Noble Topf can be a guide on your path.

The other theme is life as a labor pain. Linda regrets never having a child, but if you read her book, you will see that she gave birth to a beautiful human being—herself!

When you can see that the pain and difficulties are related to your choices and desire to live, then you will know they were all worthwhile labor pains because you can say, "I gave birth to myself." Read this book and be your own midwife to a new life.

Happy Birth Day to You!!

Bernie S. Siegel, M.D.

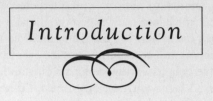

Introduction

When the heart weeps for what it has lost,
The Soul rejoices for what it has found.

Sufi expression

I n 1987, I was out walking with my six-year-old friend Jillian.
At that time I was still able to get around with a cane, but I
needed to stop quite often to rest. During one of our rest stops,
Jillian looked up and told me, "I love walking with you, Linda. I get
to see stuff when I'm with you. Most people go too fast for me. They
miss all the good stuff, you know. But you take your time."

I smiled at her simplicity and wisdom. Her words reminded me of
the changes in my life since I was first diagnosed with multiple
sclerosis. Once, my livelihood as president of one of the hottest
design/marketing shops in the nation, Noble Design Associates,

depended on my ability to perform creative perceptual shifts on a daily basis. I was considered an expert on breaking through the barriers that block creativity. My company received more than one hundred art direction and community service awards and the praise of veteran creative people worldwide for its outstanding work.

Now, as a person faced with serious illness, I'd had to make my own creative shift in order to realize that dealing with my disease meant more than simply getting rid of it. Like others in my situation, I'd discovered that with a slight shift in perception, my illness could also become a journey of self-discovery. Having accepted the current realities of my life, I found, as many others have, that choosing to make this shift could lead to a sense of wholeness that makes life better, whether the disease gets better or not. I believe there are really no real catastrophes or disasters. There is only our interpretation of events, and how we choose to interpret them helps determine how we act toward them.

In this book, I offer a perspective on loving and living successfully with illness. What I say here is not based on somebody else's good ideas, on theories, on clinical observations, or on a therapist's recommendations but on my own experience with progressive multiple sclerosis and its accompanying stress, pain, and fear. Like many others with serious, debilitating illnesses, I have embarked on a daily, moment-to-moment search for the meaning of why something like this could be happening to me. This illness has robbed me of things I have loved—dancing, running, taking steamy hot baths, tying my own shoes—even buttoning my blouse. But I have also found that there is a profoundly comforting reality beyond these losses that gives my life meaning, purpose . . . and joy.

At some point in this incredible odyssey, I asked myself, "How can I use what is happening to me as a motivator to find those answers that have allowed others before me to push aside the harsh realities of illness and find a way to live with dignity and love?" I wasn't looking to become a hero—I continue to get my greatest pleasures from a simple life—but I wanted to know what it was that made it possible for people like Helen Keller, or Franklin Roosevelt, or even Lou Gehrig to make important contributions and live full and productive lives. What could I do to use my illness as an opportunity for expansion rather than contraction, particularly when I was feeling frustrated, hopeless, and fearing that life would always be like this?

In 1984, with questions such as these in mind, I founded The MS Initiative. Through it we created a network of people who were living with this illness. We shared resources and success stories, and brought in physicians, health practitioners, and healers, some of them from mainstream medicine, others from a variety of nontraditional modes. Young and old, rich and poor, healthy and infirm, patients and their supporters of all colors and creeds came to The MS Initiative with their frustrations and joys, to gain insights on spiritual wisdom, and to share their experiences. We had rich opportunities to share what we knew with one another and to hear what people were doing at the cutting edge of medical research and the healing arts. It gave us lobbying power, to make certain our communities included facilities that allowed people in wheelchairs or with limited mobility to enjoy cultural events, concerts, lectures; to visit the parks; to go shopping or get on a bus; to enjoy a special meal in a restaurant. For five successful years, The MS Initiative became a national organization, aimed at serving others so they might know better how to live successfully with their illnesses.

My vision, and my mission, was to bring together and widely disseminate information about alternative health care and how it can help patients with MS. We had conferences where people with MS were able to experience a wide variety of health care systems firsthand. We distributed the latest information about treatment and research throughout the world.

For several years, The MS Initiative was the central focus of my life, and our membership expanded into the thousands. Through it I learned not only a great deal about my own illness, its treatment, and what therapies were available to help me be more comfortable with it, but much more than that, I experienced the deep personal fulfillment in personal relationships and inner peace that I have always enjoyed in service. I learned, in a way that would never be taken from me, that we need never be defined by illness, and it was out of the many heartening experiences with The MS Initiative and the many people I have met that I decided to write the book you are now reading.

Over the past ten years, I have counseled, lectured, and held discussion groups and seminars on spirituality and new thought. Across the United States on television and radio talk shows, I have provided encouragement to thousands and brought solace to people with life-threatening illnesses by introducing valuable keys for developing qualities of mastership as we move toward greater self-realization and spiritual enlightenment.

The message I would like to bring to anyone facing a serious illness starts with this statement: *No matter what the diagnosis, the name of the disease, or the mode of treatment, always remember that who you are is not somebody with an illness. Who you are is somebody, somebody who matters!* Embrace that somebody. Love that person. And you will discover your true identity beyond illness. This is perhaps the most important insight I have to offer others.

It is difficult to avoid approaching serious illness without negative self-judgments, anticipating tomorrow's losses or pain. Influenced by traditional conditioning, most people approach illness based only on the immediate experience of physical discomfort, fear, and deprivation. As a result, they miss out on the life-expanding experiences that are constantly being presented to those who are aware and awake enough to claim them. What I have found, with the support of my husband and best friend, Michael, my dearest friends, loved ones, and the thousands of men and women who have participated in The MS Initiative, is that there truly is another way to live with illness, one that is filled with dignity and purpose and love.

This is a how-to book, hopefully directing readers along a path for developing those traits of character that allow us to tangibly improve the quality of our lives. The anecdotes, quotes, and stories presented here are intended to help you on this journey, as you shift your perceptions and begin to find harmony and balance that you may have thought impossible up until now. The book is also intended to show supporters, caregivers, family members, and physicians a new way to relate to people with serious illness, to serve them as patients, perhaps, but more than that to establish relationships that build dignity, reducing the separation that has traditionally existed between people with illness and those who are well.

When I was first diagnosed with MS, I did not know where to turn for help. Where do we go in this world of busy specialists to find information and support for a life journey such as this? It was once assumed that we could turn to physicians, therapists, hospitals, nursing homes, schools, families, the clergy—that any or all of these might offer counsel and minister to our emotional and spiritual needs when we were confronted with this most difficult of life's challenges. Too often, the physician is a medical specialist whose knowledge is limited to what is going on in the body. The hospital

or nursing home staff is focused only on physical maintenance—
that is, meeting the basic needs of the patient. Meanwhile, family
and friends can be virtually devastated by the fact that their loved
one has a serious disease that is beyond their control. The therapist
or religious counselor may have little more than sympathy and
compassion to offer, perhaps combined with methods to ease more
serious psychological symptoms, such as depression, apathy, or loss
of faith. But where do we find the skills to make our lives full and
whole again, regardless of even the most calamitous physical losses
and symptoms? Where do we turn to reclaim dignity and purpose
and joy for ourselves?

Within traditional approaches, the person with the illness all too
often becomes an outsider in life. Personal relationships change as
we lose the ability to function in ways we once did. But in putting
the book together, I met many people who were living successfully
with serious illness, who had made peace with their lives, often in
ways they had not enjoyed prior to their illness. I met people who
had gained a level of dignity and strength that was an inspiration to
everyone around them. I met many great teachers who offered wisdom and went far beyond the old stereotypes of dealing with illness.
I found that, rather than being limiting and painful, living with
illness could be enriching. It could be, as one person has put it, a
"magnifying lens" bringing life up closer, where the truths of all
human existence, from fear to ecstasy, become better known and
better appreciated.

Most of the material in this book speaks of a journey without
doubt or hesitation, without guilt, embarrassment, or shame. In it, I
believe, is a voice that speaks to the inner part of us. To journey
through these chapters is to put oneself through a different place
and time, a time where we perceive ourselves as essentially spiritual
beings, with our central task of healing being focused on love.

The goal of this book is to help people who are living with illness
deepen their own and their loved ones' understanding of life, to
build a framework for living and loving more successfully. If the
principles, keys, and skills offered in this book achieve only that
purpose, it will have been well worth the challenge for me.

This book is intended not only as a document one reads from
cover to cover, to gather new information, but as a guide to a new
way of life, a new way of being whole with your illness. It is my
hope that you will experience what you discover here as a way to

cultivate tools and life skills that restore, renew, and strengthen you in this time of such enormous challenge.

Every writer, I suspect, hopes that his or her words will open doors for others, will offer a passage of clear light where readers can find their way. I dream that dream for this book—that it might serve as a map, charting a rich, still-to-be explored territory with vast new possibilities and new promise.

I hope that every reader will find inspiration, wisdom, and support here, awakening him or her to what is most important of all: a loving heart.

Part One

THE

ILLNESS

The day will come when,
after harnessing space, the winds, the tides, and
gravitation,
we shall harness for God the energies of love.
And on that day,
for the second time in the history of the world,
we shall have discovered fire.

Pierre Teilhard de Chardin

1

What We Feel:
The Search for
New Beginnings

*My barn having burned to the ground,
I can now see the moon.*

Japanese folk saying

If you are reading this book, the chances are that you have been recently touched by a serious illness or injury that will radically change you and your loved ones' lives. There are few events more challenging to us at so many different levels simultaneously: emotionally, financially, physically, mentally, and spiritually. Unless you have lived it yourself—as I have been doing for the past twenty-seven years—it is difficult to imagine that there really could be a way through it, a way of living successfully with a serious illness.

Through the years, I have often thought how wonderful it would be to have a mental road map, or a sort of expert travel guide, to help me find my way through this territory. It would have made the last fifteen years of living with the disabilities of multiple sclerosis not only easier but much more fulfilling and rich, helping me to move more gracefully toward enjoying my life *as it is* today. With this in mind, I have written this book, hoping it might serve others to live successfully with their illnesses. Perhaps I can help you make the breakthroughs to some of the same realizations that now bring not only normalcy but true joy into my life.

Depending on whether you are the person with the illness, a loved one of that person, or a professional caregiver who genuinely wants to better understand these life challenges, you will be reading this book from different perspectives. But my central focus throughout will be on the person with the illness.

There is a tendency when we have a crippling illness to become so identified with the disease and its treatment that we forget who we are. Always keep in mind: *we are not our illnesses*, we are still ourselves. And that is what this book is about, showing you how to reclaim your true identity in the midst of the challenge posed by critical illness.

I recently heard a man say that his illness had become a magnifier of life for him. He told me that it exaggerates everything he is, and enhances the very essence of life itself. In the process, he has been able to see himself and life much more clearly. By forcing him to look beyond everyday reality and his own mortality, he said, his illness had taken him closer to who he is, not further from himself.

I know, better than most, that illness has the potential for alienating us from ourselves. But it doesn't have to. And if this book is about nothing else, it marks out a path that will enhance and expand our lives for us—that will make it clearer who we are, bringing our true identity into focus in ways that it may be impossible for you to even imagine at this moment. I am not proposing a Pollyannaish approach to your illness, nor am I talking about positive thinking. On the contrary, the path I describe here is one that will challenge you in many ways, encouraging you to be more straightforward with yourself than is ordinarily required in everyday life. The end result will be a positive outlook and deep appreciation for who you are, sometimes not *in spite of the illness* you may have but actually *because of it*.

EMOTIONAL CHALLENGE

*Sometimes I go about pitying myself, and all the time I
am being carried on great winds across the sky.*

Chippewa saying

When we first learn that we have a serious illness, most of us are
overwhelmed by a dizzying array of emotions: fear, anger, grief, sense
of unworthiness, disappointment, guilt, despair, discouragement,
pain (both physical and emotional), and shame. This was certainly
true for me. Like the impulses of unsuspecting tourists caught in the
cross fire of a war in a foreign country, our first reflex is to do
whatever we can to escape, to flee, to hide. But of course we quickly
discover there is no place to go. Our bodies and minds, our very
souls, seem to have become both the victim and the attacker. Short
of leaving our bodies entirely, there is no escape.

Consistent with the standards of achievement that had always
guided my life, when I first accepted that I was really ill, I signed on
with experts of various sorts, each of whom promised that if I would
adhere to *this* diet, *that* vitamin, herb, regimen, or *that* physical
therapy, I would triumph over my illness.

I seized upon each explanation that doctors, nutritionists, and
various healers had to offer with the belief that, finally, this must be
the answer! Eating vegetables and brown rice is the right way!
Forget red meat. Eating raw foods and juicing vegetables is the right
way! Don't mix fruits and veggies. B_6 is good! Too much is bad.
Eating protein in strict food combinations is the right way! Eat more
fish, but look out for fish oils. Watch out for shellfish. A high-
protein diet is the best. B_{12} shots are a must! Eating by rotating food
families is the right way! Beware of transfatty acids in margarine. Eat
red meat. Fasting for twenty-four hours once a week is the right way.

Intramuscular injections of "live cells" in Tijuana, Mexico, snake
venom oil, phenol injections in my legs, aquatic therapy, homeopa-
thy, raw vegetable juicing, weekly colonic irrigations, ceremonial
rituals, sweat lodges and living with the Lakota in South Dakota,
deep muscle massage, chi energy balancing, hyperbaric oxygen,
ground ginseng root, a myriad of detoxification programs, daily en-
zymes and food supplements, MRIs, a lacto-vegetarian diet, a macro-

biotic diet, chemical sensitivities, mercury amalgam temporal removal, distilled water, electric magnetic field testing, chiropractic treatment and kinesiology, acupuncture, energy work, Kombucha "tea" mushrooms, and now, Beta interferon. The more determined I was, the more confused I became. Finally, I threw up my hands! "I don't know," I said. "I don't know that anyone has the answer I am seeking! Perhaps there really is no escape."

As terrifying as this realization was, there was a very positive, though at first quite puzzling, revelation that came out of it. I learned that the discovery that there is no escape can become a real blessing, and a gift. The moment we accept the fact that there is no escape, we begin living much more in the present. We begin to take life in, truly absorb it at its most essential. We discover how even our fondest dreams and aspirations, for all the good that is in them, also have a way of insulating us from ourselves.

I remember going in for an appointment to see a neurologist in Philadelphia. On this day I was feeling particularly sad and hopeless about my situation. During the medical consultation, I broke down and cried, "Why is God abandoning me? Why has he forgotten me?" The doctor, intuitive and wise, having witnessed many others going through what I was only beginning to struggle with, replied, "Linda, God has not abandoned you. He has chosen you."

*When the gods choose to punish us,
they merely answer our prayers.*

Oscar Wilde

I am not going to tell you that I immediately understood what he was saying, because I didn't. At this point, God was the furthest thing from my mind. The God that I knew was *punishing* me, not *choosing* me.* However, since I recognized that he knew something I didn't, what he'd said stayed in my mind, a constant reminder

* I will use the word God throughout the book interchangeably with other expressions, such as Spirit, the Light, I AM, Source, Higher Self, Oneness, Inner Guidance, Inner Voice, Wholeness, Essence, or Love, to describe the spiritual aspect of who we are, always referring to the source of love existing within all of us. (It doesn't matter what you call this sustaining energy I call God.) As this is a very individual and personal matter, I encourage you to see what fits for you.

that perhaps there truly was another way of looking at my challenge.

Even knowing that there were alternatives to what I was thinking and feeling, denial, the powerful mechanism that takes over in us all at critical times, screamed out, *"This cannot be happening to me!"* It was my first line of defense against my fear. No doubt about it, denial can be a blessed buffer, softening the blow. It buys us a little time while we learn how we are going to manage the rest of our lives. But if we pay very close attention to how this protective reflex affects us overall, we soon discover that denial also has its downside.

As contradictory as it may seem to us, the fact is that denial can never liberate us from our fear or bring us anything like lasting comfort. On the contrary, as we learn to accept the fact that there is no escape, we begin moving beyond our fear and emotional turmoil; we begin *acknowledging* our emotions. We begin to live, whether we have an illness or not, the moment we stop *denying* or trying to run from our emotions. Surprising as it might seem, those difficult emotions we all spend so much of our lives trying to escape are not the enemy at all *but the light that can guide us out of the darkness.*

The temptation, however, is to argue that with all the other problems we're faced with—be it physical pain, financial pressures, family upheaval—we haven't got time to deal with emotions. I know. I have been there myself and discovered that in spite of all the other challenges, our own feelings about our illness are at the center of all other issues we are facing. And how we address those most difficult emotions will determine whether we reclaim ourselves, and live our lives successfully, or sacrifice our very souls to the illness.

The Diagnosis

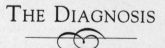

Death is not the greatest loss in life, the greatest loss is
what dies inside us while we live.

Norman Cousins

The first struggle most of us have comes immediately after hearing the fateful diagnosis. For me, it began at the University of Pennsylvania Hospital, with the terse, stoic neurologist who gave my husband, Michael, and me the diagnosis. I was terribly frightened and terribly naïve about what was happening to me, yet perhaps out of that I became quite assertive, asking even this unsympathetic physician many questions. *What exactly was happening to my legs?* I wanted to know. *Where could I gather additional information? What could I do now?* The reply I got wasn't the one I had anticipated or would have wanted. The doctor leaned toward us, ignoring my desperate questions, and to my surprise and revulsion said, "Too bad you're so cute. You'll be in a wheelchair, you know! You might as well go home and wait. There is nothing you can do."

His cruel insensitivity triggered something deep within me, and I didn't hold back. I remember glaring at him, snapping, "You have no idea who you are talking to, buddy!" I stormed out of his office deeply upset and depressed. In hindsight, I see this doctor unwittingly activated *my will to live* in the face of serious illness.

In the beginning, my own intense denial of my illness, and how it would have an impact on my life in the years ahead, was accompanied by an explosive rage, welling up from deep within me. That rage eventually unleashed my strength, my courage, my ability to survive, and my passion to make a positive difference in the world. But first I had to acknowledge my anger fully to myself. Instead of raging against the parts of my life that could not be changed, I began to take a new look at my life's priorities, carefully selecting what was truly important to me. I began to rebuild my self-image, seeing that life is much more than the past goals, achievements, and expectations by which I had judged myself.

I have always been a survivor, something I learned at an early age. That pattern was set. Especially now, I couldn't give that up. Those qualities of determination that served me in my earliest life now enabled me to go forward, to explore how I might live successfully with illness. The courage and tenacity that I had learned as a child now prepared me to enter this new and totally foreign world in which I would slowly and painfully lose many of my physical capacities.

For many months, I was devastated, terrified at the prospect of a life of limited mobility. I felt like damaged goods. Perhaps like you, I had never considered the possibility of being the one who would have a life-threatening illness. Surely, there had to be a mistake. "Not me!" I cried desperately. "I'm getting ready to begin my life!"

I wanted to have children. I wanted to travel. I wanted the best art studio in the country. I wanted to run a marathon. I had my dreams! And now, now . . . I couldn't believe it . . . not only would I be unable to dance, an activity in which I'd once taken particular delight, but before long I wouldn't even be able to walk! Inside, I cried, *Don't take these from me! I want to live!*

Left to my own devices, with emotional support from my dear husband, Michael, I became my own authority figure. No disease was going to determine the course of my life! For years I simply shoved back my feelings of loss, living as if nothing was ever *really* going to change. I numbed myself to my fears. I focused on selling my artwork, on photography, on advertising, on graphic design, on marketing, on public relations, on writing. I just *assumed* I would succeed at whatever I chose, because I knew how to manipulate the system.

Along with all my denial, I began to close myself off from those around me. After all, how would I ever dare let other people know what I would not even tell myself! I worried constantly about revealing myself. I was reluctant to risk any kind of closeness or intimacy, feeling that if people found out about my illness it would end the relationship or put both of us in an agonizing double bind between love and the fear of the disease. I was certain all this would drive apart any friendships and business relationships I might try to foster. I lived every day with a heartbreaking mixture of vulnerability and toughness.

However, as successful as I was at hiding from the truth, there were times when it all came rushing in on me, the flood of reality producing huge waves of emotion paralyzing in their effect. In my worst moments, I felt like a complete failure—a failure in fulfilling my dreams, my talent, a physical failure, unable to save my body from this horrible disease that was ravaging it. I felt I had let myself down, and was surely letting down those who loved me. I was caught up in a whirlwind of thoughts and feelings, of self-blame, despair, judgment, sense of unworthiness, panic, destruction, and isolation. I had this need to prove myself over and over again, because I was never quite good enough in my own eyes.

Around those who looked up to me or who looked to me for strength, I put up a good front. But inside, I secretly lived with a constantly nagging sense of failure—that I was going to be found out—that I was an impostor, knowing that my tough exterior only masked a crumbling interior. I had always taken such pride in my independence! I had always done everything myself, and now I was losing control of my life and the ability to do things that I had always valued so highly. Issues of dependency, such as the prospect of having to ask other people to help me dress or go to the bathroom, overwhelmed me. I felt desperate, scared, and very, very sorry for myself.

I lived with these inner conflicts, denials, and fears for years. And along with all the other emotions I was fighting, a new one began to emerge and grow: my anger. Every time I stopped to think about the reality of the doctor's diagnosis, I would start feeling that my whole life was being wrenched away. With this feeling I discovered the real depth of my anger. My disease was robbing me of everything I held dear. In my fury, I began to hate anyone who was well, who was sound of body. I did that for a long time, until I discovered another side of this emotion we call anger. When I examined it very closely, I discovered that hidden within my anger was a powerful and abiding *will to live*. And I saw that it was possible to get beyond my negative expressions of this emotion and actually embrace the positive side of it, thus tapping into an inner resource that might otherwise have eluded me forever.

EMBRACE YOUR WILL TO LIVE

People are always blaming their circumstances for what they are. I don't believe in circumstances. The people who get on in this world are the people who get up and look for the circumstances they want, and, if they can't find them, make them.

George Bernard Shaw

I am not certain when I began to change. But one incident in particular stands out. Michael and I were driving along the Pennsylvania Turnpike when I suddenly had to go to the bathroom. The first stop we came to was a fast-food restuarant. This was no time to be choosy. We raced into the parking lot, quickly assembled my electric scooter and I sped into the restaurant in search of the bathroom. Once inside, I was faced with the embarrassing task of having to ask a total stranger for help. Michael could not help me, of course, because it was a public rest room, for women only.

It took all the courage I had at the moment to overcome my sense of humiliation and tell the man at the counter that I needed help in the bathroom— and I needed it immediately. He beckoned a young dark-haired woman who was bussing dishes. She dutifully followed along behind me, holding the door to the bathroom for me as I scooted into the tiny, tiled room. When we got inside I soon discovered that my helper didn't speak English, and I didn't speak Spanish, which turned out to be her native tongue.

Somehow, through hand signals and body language, we managed to communicate with each other enough to get me on the toilet. I then asked her to give me some privacy but to come back soon. She left, returning within a minute or two with a glass of ice water. As she held out the glass of water for me to take from her, I stared at her in disbelief, my incredulity mixed with frustration, humiliation, and anger. This glass of ice water seemed so totally inappropriate! What could she be thinking of!

A part of me wanted to lash out at her, to make her the target of all the anger I felt—at the difficulty of finding a wheelchair-accessible bathroom in the first place, at the embarrassment I had to go through just to take care of such a basic physical necessity, and above all in having a body that would not do my bidding. But in that moment, something very important shifted within me. I saw that perhaps I actually had a choice about the way I looked at the world around me. I found, beyond my anger, this awkward encounter in the bathroom of a fast-food restaurant on the turnpike became an opportunity to see life very differently than I otherwise would have. It suddenly dawned on me what the most immediate problem was. And by focusing on it, rather than on all the problems around my physical condition, I felt the emotional distance between me and my helper dissolve. Apparently, something I said might have led her to bring me ice water. However, I believe it was ultimately her compassion and generosity that bridged the language gap.

Suddenly I saw the humor in all of it and I laughed out loud. Here I was, on an obstacle course of ramps that challenged me to defy gravity, wrestling with heavy doors, maneuvering around curb cuts placed directly in front of parking places so that there was no room to get through in my wheelchair. And then there was this rest room, located one flight down from the dining room, and I was unable even to go to the bathroom by myself, forced to ask for help from total strangers.

As if that wasn't enough, my helper and I couldn't communicate verbally because we spoke two different languages. Clearly, I was surrounded by obstacles that indeed had the potential for creating a lot of frustration. But the total absurdity of it somehow helped open my eyes to my own humanness and to the kindness of this young woman who really was doing her very best to be helpful. Somewhere in all of that was a lesson, an insight that allowed me to begin taking a fresh look at the meaning of my life. In spite of our mutual awkwardness, there was something very touching and precious and valuable about the moment. In our bumbling, clumsy, embarrassed efforts to attend to the most basic and elemental of human necessities, our hearts had joined.

As Michael and I got back into the car and sped on our way, I recognized that something important had happened back there. I had been able to see my life beyond my thoughts, judgments, expectations, and beliefs, breaking apart the presuppositions that had come to rule my life, shaping my feelings and my actions. I felt almost ecstatic, recognizing that this awareness provided me with a freedom that was indeed profound and heartwarming.

USE EVERYTHING TO YOUR ADVANTAGE

God speaks to all individuals through what happens to them moment by moment.

J. P. de Caussade

I had never thought of it this way before, but I began to see that it is our own perceptions that imprison us. Most of the time, it really does appear that the way we see the world is the way the world really is—and there is no other way to look at it. We find it difficult to see our perceptions for what they are—an inner movie about the way life "ought" to be. It isn't easy to see that we ourselves are creating the way we experience life, forcing it into our own molds, judging it against the inner movie instead of taking life in as it really is. The incident in the bathroom, breaking through my own perceptions to connect in a loving way with the woman who was trying to help me, allowed me to see that we have a choice not only about how we relate to events around us but how we relate to ourselves and to the perceptions we hold in our minds.

At first it wasn't easy to hold on to this rather complex realization. I must confess that there are still many times when it eludes me and I fall back into the old patterns. But the more I exercise this option in my life, the easier it gets, and the more I am able to be free of my perceptions of how life *should be,* opening up a space to find another way of looking at the world. This is the real healing for all of us, able-bodied or not, a freeing up of the illusions of life so that we can step squarely into the process of what our lives are really about: living successfully with the way *it is.*

CRISIS AS OPPORTUNITY

What concerns me is not the way things are, but rather the way people think things are.

Epictetus

Out of the awkward bathroom episode, I began to feel that life itself—so often unveiled to us in our least graceful moments—was important and valuable and precious to me. And I knew that this outlook was what I needed to pursue in my healing. Though I continued to do everything possible to regain my physical health, I began to catch the first glimpses of the insight that would give me a brand-new way to live my life. The first priority in the healing I sought wasn't so much a matter of restoring my physical body to health but of learning to live life successfully, regardless of my diagnosis or my physical condition.

This insight was, of course, filled with contradictions whose resolutions would unfold only slowly, and in some very unexpected ways. I think the first step was to look at my life, and the lives of others in similar situations, and ask myself a question that at first seemed quite odd: *"What is the true meaning of the word health?"*

By all definitions, I am not physically healthy. But if I have learned nothing else from my illness, it is that health can not be defined in terms of one's physical condition. This single realization allowed me to suddenly take a quantum leap beyond my denial into an acceptance wherein I literally began to reclaim my life. I realized that true *quality of life* can never be found by avoiding suffering. As I got to know others who'd faced challenges similar to mine, and observed those who were living full lives even though they were obviously suffering from extremely debilitating illnesses, it became clear to me that *being healed isn't the same as being cured of one's illness*. For me, this realization has posed as many new questions as answers. What exactly was it that needed to be healed in order to live successfully with this disease? Surely there had to be another way of looking at my life, one that would allow me to live to the fullest, regardless of my diagnosis, and regardless of what apparent limitations my illness seemed to impose.

In the beginning, my sense of powerlessness over the disease, my sense of this mysterious illness taking over my body and robbing me of the physical capacities I'd always taken so much for granted, filled me with frustration, fear, and anger. Episodes such as the one in the bathroom, which I described earlier, convinced me that above all I did not want these feelings to become the center of my life. But what choice did I have? Certainly, to be expected to be immune to such feelings in the face of the extreme physical discomfort associated with catastrophic illness wasn't the answer. One didn't have to be a genius to figure that one out!

In reflecting back over my own experiences, it is my observation that the absence of anger in the face of a serious illness suggests that we have already withdrawn from life, that we have relinquished our passion for living, that we are resigned and emotionally numb. So, in spite of the fact that our society teaches us that anger is "negative," my advice to people seeking another way of looking at their life is to not think badly of yourself for feeling angry. On the contrary, think of it as a resource that you can learn to harness and refine for your own benefit. As you begin to *own* your anger, which we'll be talking more about as we go along, you'll discover how it can help you reclaim your personal identity.

It is not easy to admit to our anger. After all, there is pain, regret, and fear in it. But when we do find a way to acknowledge it, one that feels safe for us, we start to live again, experiencing the full breadth of our emotions, from grief and anger to joy and compassion, and from resentment and jealousy to empathy and love. In the process many people fully embrace life for the very first time, illness or not. As difficult as this process was at the time, I sometimes catch myself wondering if I might otherwise never have gotten in touch with what is truly magical about my life—and, believe me, there is much that I find truly joyous, illness or not.

I can now say, without a shadow of doubt, that when we get in touch with our anger and fully acknowledge it as our own, we find that it holds treasures that previously had been quite impossible to see. We discover that it is first and foremost a demand for change. In this respect it is very often the way we initially open up to experience our true nature, *the spiritual self*. When we allow anger, we look beyond our perceptions and move forward to discover the preciousness of our lives.

Helplessness, frustration, and anger are not the only difficult emotions that surface with serious illness. We may also find ourselves filled with blame, looking for someone or something to punish, or seeking ways to blame and punish ourselves. There are those with critical injuries that make it difficult or impossible for them to function on a physical level, whose fate was the result of their own poor judgment or the poor judgment of others. When faced with such truths, it is difficult to get past the blame because there really does appear to be a person or persons responsible for the injury. However, unless we let go of the blame seeker in ourselves, we will forever be held hostage by our own bitterness.

Don't get me wrong. Like anger and frustration, blame is bound to arise when we're faced with serious illness or injury. There are still times when I blame myself for being sick; for not having children; for cancelling vacations; for not being able to run on the beach; for needing to travel with a scooter in airports, on the streets, in art museums, and in shopping malls; for having small, spindly veins that are difficult to take blood from; for feeling unproductive and for defining *unproductive* as failing to be worthy in anyone's eyes —particularly my own. Since I am a person who has always been focused on what I could accomplish in a day, it has been very difficult to get beyond the belief that my worth as a human being could be measured by what I produce in a day.

The self-blame I experienced in this regard began to diminish only when I recognized it as anger—*my anger*. This anger, in turn, derived from my *perception* that one's worth could be measured only in terms of productivity. There was a great sense of freedom that came when I recognized this. I realized that while I might not be able to change the physical reality of my illness, I could change the perceptions I held in my own mind. Paradoxically, however, it was only through fully owning the anger I was experiencing that this became possible.

STILL HUMAN, STILL WHOLE

Courage is mastery of fear, not absence of fear.

Mark Twain

Most people with serious illnesses, such as the ones we're addressing in this book, must come to terms with a sense of being separated from the whole human race. When I first began this odyssey, and particularly when the symptoms of my illness made it impossible to do things I'd once found so easy and rewarding to do, I felt like a complete outsider in life. This sense of alienation and separation from others also took place in my relationships with other people; as my physical abilities diminished, it became increasingly obvious to me that I was different from them—at least, that's how it looked on the surface. They moved about freely on their own two feet, while I found it difficult, and finally impossible, to move my legs enough to even put on my own socks; I required an electric scooter to get around, and needed help just to get in and out of cars. All these things seemed to be proof of how different I was from other people, and out of the sense of these differences it was easy to conclude that I really felt cut off from the rest of the human race.

Often, I felt as though I was looking at the world through dark, distorted glasses—as it says in the Bible, "Now I look through a glass darkly." I could see other people, and knew they could see me, but I felt as if I somehow couldn't touch them or be with them. I felt that people didn't want to listen and couldn't ever understand my life experience. We seemed of two different cultures entirely— the physically healthy and the unhealthy! This sense of isolation, of being separate from people who are well, can be as painful as any of the worst treatments or symptoms that we might have to endure. It is loneliness in its most profound form. Though this loneliness, too, is the product of our own perceptions, it is one of the most difficult to grasp and the most challenging to let go of.

Many philosophers, psychologists, and spiritual leaders have said that being human is lonely whether we have an illness or not. Still, I firmly believe that there is a natural process that moves us all toward wholeness, drawing us together so that we can find and experience our oneness. I am now convinced that my illness guided me to better appreciate that process, to look beyond the surface of physical attributes, beliefs, and even feelings, to get in touch with that part of each and every one of us that is the spiritual nucleus of all life. I won't lie about it; I would have preferred to come to these insights by some other path. But there is no denying that through the challenge of illness I've received a deeper understanding of my vulnerability, a greater openness than I might ever have otherwise known. It allowed me to discover the spiritual reality of my life, the place in our hearts we all share, where we are all joined as one. I can honestly say my illness helped me discover the gift of my humanness and wholeness in a way that might otherwise have remained hidden from me forever.

PERCEPTION AS INTERPRETATION

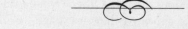

What lies behind us and what lies before us are small matters compared to what lies within us.

Ralph Waldo Emerson

The key to these changes is within everyone's grasp. It is a matter of recognizing that our own perceptions about what life "should be" are not fixed, not carved in granite, but are like movies playing in our minds and projecting out into life. Our healing comes when we realize this and recognize that the movie (perception) we are projecting out onto the world is only one vision in an infinite number that we might choose to make. And we truly can choose. We can choose to rewrite our "inner movie" scripts, thus changing our perceptions, and provide ourselves with a very different interpretation of our reality, one where our lives are meaningful and whole regardless of our illness or apparent physical limitations.

When we let ourselves be open to the possibility that there might be another way of looking at our lives, beyond our own present perceptions of what life *should be*, we soon find ourselves discovering realities where even our worst fears are comforted and soothed. We discover that the loneliness we have so often experienced, which naturally grows out of the wound those like us suffer, can open us to the healing and love all around us, which has always been all around us, though we could not see. There is a way that our diseases can ultimately propel us forward, appreciating and enjoying our humanness more than ever. And in a very real way, that is what this book is about, about sharing with others what we can do to get in touch with our humanness and the strengths and joys we may not have even guessed we possess.

When we have a serious illness, it's a great challenge to learn to trust life again. Suddenly, we feel all too vulnerable, fragile, and perhaps fragmented. But every time I meet another patient who has learned to live successfully with his or her illness—and there are a great many—I am once again inspired to trust life, even when things are looking very bleak. I trust the ability for each one of us to deal with our own pain, fear, and grief, to transcend our loneliness and become more in touch with who we are and the spirit within us. Every one of us is wounded, whether or not we have been diagnosed as having a serious disease. Others' wounds may not be as obvious as ours, may not appear to have as dramatic an impact on their lives as ours, but they are definitely there. What's more, the process for healing is always the same and is available for all of us.

What We Really Wish to Heal

Never give in. Never. Never. Never. Never.

Winston Churchill

When I first was diagnosed with MS, I ran out and bought hundreds of dollars' worth of books about how to gain control over this disease. That was my first effort to regain a sense of being in charge of my life, the only way I immediately saw to possibly trust life again. Without the hope of gaining mastery over this disease, I believed life was hardly worth living.

Many of the books I read and "experts" I spoke to talked about how love, forgiveness, joy, and optimism are positive emotions, while sadness, fear, and anger are negative. Many also said that the negative emotions are dangerous, that they are to be avoided, that if we do allow ourselves to experience these feelings, the illness will get worse. But it has been my experience that suppressing or denying these emotions is where the real dangers lie. Keeping these emotions bottled up or covering them up with "positive affirmations" takes a huge amount of energy and ultimately is the source of additional stress in our lives. Our healing begins when we acknowledge these feelings to ourselves, not in a way that might be hurtful (to others or ourselves), but simply when we acknowledge, in a gentle way, that they are there.

I have to say that, in the beginning, avoiding negative emotions seemed to make sense to me. But what has proved to be more to the point is that there are no "bad" or negative emotions. In many respects, our emotions are the very essence of human life; to deny them—whether positive or negative—is to deny life itself. All emotions engage us with life, and it is through this engagement that we learn to trust life again. In that respect, all our emotions are positive and potentially life-affirming.

What I have discovered for myself is that we cannot avoid our negative emotions if we hope to live successfully with illness. On the contrary, we must open up to them. When we undergo an injury or illness that radically alters the way we live, which forces us to change our dreams, aspirations, and expectations of our lives, there is no doubt about it—one of the most intense and disturbing things we're going to experience is our sense of loss. And these losses will trigger a lot of frustration, feelings of helplessness, and anger, all of which can be very scary. When we open up to our negative feelings, and acknowledge the emotional loss and pain, we begin the process of *self-acceptance*—an essential step toward changing our perceptions and living successfully with an illness. To deny that we are angry for having the lives we have known torn from us is to create separation and alienation from the very things in life we hold most dear. In addition, that denial prevents us from identifying and letting go of our old perceptions of what life is all about and opening up to how we are going to live successfully with our illness from this day forward. The inner healing that we seek comes not in our denial but in our surrendering to the truth, to *life as it is*.

Acknowledging these realities can be painful, to be sure. However, in taking on that challenge, we give ourselves another chance to love life again, regardless of the physical, emotional, and mental pain we may be experiencing. I have often heard it said that wherever there is mental and emotional pain, "the only way out is through." In other words, instead of denying or avoiding our pain, we need to plunge into the middle of it, not in a careless and impulsive way but with guidance and understanding. When we learn to open our hearts and minds, the guidance and understanding come from many sources, from others as well as ourselves. With open hearts we discover that we are never alone and that the changes we are seeking are as close as a thought.

In my own life I discovered that allowing myself to experience my negative emotions, something very unexpected occurred: instead of the negative feelings increasing, they actually diminished. As I drew closer to them, no longer denying or suppressing them, I began to feel much more positive about my life. It was like taking the pressure out of the pressure cooker. Suddenly, I had much more energy and I felt as if huge blocks of time opened up to me when I could thoroughly enjoy my life.

Life Skill #1

Whenever negative thoughts, fears, judgments, and self-blame arise in your mind, challenge them. Acknowledge that they are not facts, no matter how much "justification" you may find for them. Let yourself be guided by the belief that there is another way of looking at your life, and then be determined to find it.

CHOOSING WHAT TO DISCARD

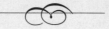

Fall seven times, stand up eight.

Japanese proverb

If we are to live successfully with a serious illness, we really must reexamine many facets of our lives beyond our physical concerns. And in the process we may find much that needs to be discarded because it no longer serves us. I am still letting go of behaviors, emotional attachments, and habit patterns that no longer serve me well. For example, I once believed that we need to get our lives more *in order* to be whole. But I have discovered that healing comes when I put *less emphasis on the order* that I would impose on the world and *more emphasis on expressions* that come from acceptance, love, and the simplicity of the heart.

REDEFINING HELPLESSNESS

As we discover beliefs and dreams that no longer serve us, and as we make the decisions to let them go, there is no way to avoid experiencing a sense of loss. Ironically, we can even experience a sense of loss when choosing to let go of something that causes us pain or that we know does not serve us well. So, learning to deal with loss is itself an important part of living successfully with serious illness. Whether we are well or ill, there is no way to be alive and avoid the pain of loss. It's all part of life, just as our feelings of anger and blame are a part of life.

For most people, the loss of independence is one of the most challenging aspects of having a serious illness. One of the ways I first experienced this was in dressing myself. As healthy adults with able bodies, we take this simple act for granted. Maybe when I was a child I didn't give a second thought to getting help with my clothes, but the forty-five-year-old in me still says, at my age I should at least be able to tie my shoelaces in the morning! It still startles me and makes me very sad when I have to ask for help getting dressed or have to ask for help crossing or uncrossing my legs as I struggle to put my socks on. With the muscles in my legs in spasm, I can't put my shoes on, let alone my underpants!

We don't easily give up these areas of independence. To be perfectly honest, it still surprises me when I am pushed to confront my feelings about this. I find myself trying to act strong, but the more I do that, the more distant I feel from those who are there to help. So, I don't buy button-down blouses or clothing with complicated construction. With elastic waistbands on my pants and Velcro fasteners, I've at least made it easy for others to help me, but I have to say that it has not reduced my awareness of how much help I need. I try to make it as easy as possible on myself and those who help me in the bathroom or who assist me in getting dressed in the morning. I do my best to consider others at a handicapped rest room or in any situation where I would need to accept challenging circumstances with a minimum of embarrassment for myself and my helpers.

All these details are part of the whole picture, of course. But they are only the most obvious changes we must make if we wish to live successfully with our physical challenges. At their core are issues that are a little tougher to address—issues of independence, of being dependent on others to meet even our most basic needs.

This morning, when I began writing this, Michael was just leaving for a week-long business trip to California. As he was preparing to leave, I looked at my feelings of loss around his departure. I certainly didn't feel free at that moment. I certainly didn't feel I was in charge of my life! As I anticipated his leaving, I felt scared. Certainly, there was some justification for me to be concerned. What would I do if there was an emergency, such as a fire in the house? What would I do if something went wrong with my electric scooter and I couldn't get around? But there was another level of loss that I discovered I was feeling. I was feeling a loss because I once loved being alone. I enjoyed doing things by myself. Now, I can't remember the last time I was without constant aid—someone to spend the night, somebody to do for me what I had once enjoyed doing for myself. As Michael and I kissed good-bye and he raced off to catch his plane, I had to admit that I was afraid to be by myself. I was afraid something might happen that I'd not be able to handle. I had to come to terms with the fact that I was extremely vulnerable when I was alone.

These fears, of course, are not unfounded, as anyone with serious illness knows. After Michael left, I was alone for an hour or two and had to get to the bathroom quickly. The muscles in my legs went into spasm, and I couldn't turn my electric scooter on fast enough. I figured, well, I could just go in my pants, and that wouldn't be the worst thing or the first time. Or I could call my next-door neighbor.

Finally, I chose to call my neighbor. Gail came rushing over and helped me pull down my pants. Her presence quieted my rattled nerves. I felt embarrassed and yet I was inspired by my familiar *will to survive*, recognizing that I had reached out for help without blaming myself or feeling insecure or trying to act stronger or more independent than I really am.

COPING WITH LOSS

What you are afraid of overtakes you.

Estonian proverb

For a person with an illness like mine, coping with loss becomes a daily issue. One day I am faced with the possibility of never being able to use my left foot again. Another day I am faced with not being able to put on my underwear or my socks by myself. Another time, I discover that I can no longer cross my legs, balance a heavy mug of tea, talk on a public pay phone, climb stairs, walk into my shower, stand for two minutes, or give Michael a "stand-up" hug. Bit by bit, I have faced the loss of some of life's most common experiences—legibly signing my name or taking hot baths, for example. I never know if I will get worse today, tonight, tomorrow morning, or at noon. And there are times when the loss is bigger than any of these—when I lose myself and become just another person with multiple sclerosis, a woman with a label and no real life.

Issues of loss, strength and weakness, dependence and independence touch all of us, whether we are well or ill. How do we come to terms with loss? How do we find the truth beyond our losses that will make us free! For me, these are no longer questions so much as

exclamations. Yet, I must say that it is often on my worst days—
that is, days when I am confronted with the most painful losses—
that I have the biggest breakthroughs.

In learning to cope with loss, it is essential to learn that we must
focus not on the object or the function we are losing but on our
perception of the loss, on our interpretation of what it means. We
may have no choice about what we are losing, but we do have some
choice about how we interpret that loss. It is important to always
remember that we are in charge of our perceptions of our lives. And
whether we are a super athlete challenging world records or a person
in a wheelchair with only minimal physical capacities, it is our
perceptions that will either imprison us or set us free. To discover
that we have a choice about our perceptions, that there is a way to
shift them so that our lives can be whole, regardless of our physical
condition, is one of the most liberating breakthroughs any of us can
ever have.

Whenever I need inspiration and encouragement, I recall the
film *My Left Foot,* about Christy Brown, an Irish writer and artist
with cerebral palsy who wrote and painted with his left foot, the
only part of him over which he had much control. This true story
never ceases to remind me of the capacity of the human spirit,
which flourishes when we surrender to the way life is, refusing to be
limited by our perceptions about how life *should be*.

While working on this book, I developed a new tremor in my left
hand. It prevented me from writing, from typing, from carrying a
glass of water, and from painting, which I'd always dearly loved. I
remembered Auguste Renoir, with crippling arthritis, strapping
brushes to his hands and painting with longer, more fluid strokes, to
create some of his best works. Also, Henry Matisse, confined to bed
in his later life and unable to work with paints; instead, he created
huge, stunning compositions from colored papers, cut out with scis-
sors, as he lay in bed.

And so, I record what I wish to say on audio cassettes, which
Eunice, my typist, transcribes. I am learning to paint with watercol-
ors, no longer trying to prevent my hand from trembling but using
the trembling to create rhythmic strokes of color and movement
that somehow depict *life the way it really is*. The result is tender and
sweet, reminding me of beautiful Japanese calligraphic paintings.

When life throws you a curve, it's to teach you
how to bend.

Anonymous

One by one, my perceptions of my life have made themselves known to me in ways that I could not deny. I came to recognize, for example, that most of my life I had measured my self-worth by what I could physically accomplish in a day. *What I did* was who I was. I defined myself by my monthly calendar of goals and how well I accomplished them. But there came a time when I literally collided with this perception of myself. I saw that if that continued to be the only way I could determine my sense of self-worth, I had to ask, "Who am I now, when I can't even walk up the stairs?"

I quickly saw that who I really am is someone more than a person who can no longer walk up stairs or who is becoming less and less able to accomplish certain other tasks in the physical world. Who I am is someone who cannot be validated through my old measurements—that is to say, my old perceptions of self-worth based on accomplishment.

In my quest for a deeper understanding of who I am, beyond my perceptions—who I am beyond this person who is daily losing physical capacities that most people take for granted—I can't deny that there are many mornings when I wake up with an acute sense of loss. And there are nights when I lie awake, staring at the ceiling, searching for some explanation of what is going on and why I have gotten this illness. Why would God let this happen to me? The answers have often come in the most unexpected ways, and paradoxically they have always amazed me and lightened my heart, bringing me a new appreciation for my life.

I have always believed that the truth will set us free. And I still very much believe that. But as liberating as the truth can be, it can also be pretty frightening when it comes to loss. How can we look upon truth as *freeing* at those times when it means accepting further loss, when it means giving up dreams that we now know can never come true? What possibly can motivate us to seek the truth when it is very clear that doing so is going to produce more loss and take away things that have given us great pleasure?

Certainly, if we are to give up our early measures of our self-worth, particularly if they are based on physical accomplishment, we must find another way of looking at our lives. We all know, deep in our hearts, that a human being is much more than his or her achievements in the physical world. But what more is there? What can we turn to as new sources of fulfillment when all the old ways of winning self-worth have been wrenched from us?

Inevitably, those of us who struggle with serious physical illnesses discover that the real healing we are seeking may have little if anything to do with our bodies. In fact, it comes with our realization of a higher purpose, a part of each of us that is beyond physical loss, and beyond the restrictions we impose on our lives through our perceptions.

In private, in meditation, in support groups, I have found little glimpses of the reality that lie beyond those measurements of self-worth that no longer apply to my life. I know that my true identity cannot be found in my body or in my accomplishments in the external world; I am not my flesh and bones. I am a child of God, and God adores me. It is with this realization in mind that I have learned to cope with my worldly losses. My prayer has been "May I become more radiant than my external self."

Beyond our identification with the physical world and our accomplishments in it, there emerges for many of us the awareness that who we are is a light from beyond this world, a spiritual essence that has very little to do with the physical world of doctor appointments, medication, how we feel, what we earn, what we believe, sports results, our latest promotion at work, our education, our hair, clothes, and makeup.

Life Skill #2

Begin a personal journal. Use it to express yourself and to record feelings and insights that come up as you read this book. It is also a good place to record your thoughts and your work on the exercises as you go along. I encourage you to be as creative as you like, writing down single insights, feelings, symbols, dreams, plans, inspirational quotes, poems, and ideas that come out of the blue. Try colored pens and pencils, inserting photos or other graphic material whenever these might seem relevant to you.

Our healing often begins when we realize that we are ultimately responsible for how we see ourselves. We can choose to see our spiritual essence or to see ourselves only in terms of our illness. For example, in our culture we are bombarded by judgments of those who are ill or physically challenged as inferior, deformed, or even "wrong." At some point, we cannot help but incorporate this kind of thinking into our own set of perceptions about life. As a result we judge ourselves just as others would judge us. It is only from an enlightened spiritual perspective that we can reclaim our true glory. When we are aware of our spiritual essence, a thin, spindly vein or a leg spasm or a bulky electric scooter are all irrelevant, just not that big a deal.

But how do we get to the point of healing ourselves in this way? How do we change the perceptions that prevent us from seeing our true identity, our radiance? Healing begins with a decision to change and a willingness to accept God's help. For many of us, this requires a significant change of mind; for others, it is the most natural expression in the world. As we shift our perceptions toward our spiritual essence, we can no longer believe in the power of loss, fear, and grief that so often appears to dominate our daily lives. It is this shift in consciousness, from denial to acceptance to personal freedom, that separates the lost and disconnected patients from those who love and live successfully with their illness.

As we accept God's help in our healing, we move closer and closer to Spirit, closer and closer to the love deep inside ourselves. As we come to this spiritual perspective, our perceptions of loss are altered.

Our spiritual essence is non-material, non-physical, nonintellectual, and non-emotional. As we become aware of this, we come to see the truth as God created it, not as we have made it. We begin to see the truth beyond our own limited perceptions, and beyond our interpretations of the world and our role in it. And the more this occurs, the less we fall prey to false hopes, to the fears and losses by which we measure ourselves in the physical world. From this perspective, we embrace the source of love and healing within each of us. We begin to get in touch with our humanness and the strength we may have only prayed we might possess.

Thus, while I am not saying not to do everything you can to maintain physical well-being, I am saying that our true healing occurs beyond the physical, mental, and emotional levels. The ultimate healing might mean letting go of any investment in the physical outcome. "Thy will be done" means just that—*Thy will*, not *our will*. As I seek the truth in my life, the path before me unfolds, and I find myself moving closer to Spirit in a very peaceful, natural way.

PERCEPTUAL HEALING
IN EVERYDAY LIFE

Love alone is capable of uniting living beings in such a way as to complete and fulfill them, for it alone takes them and joins them by what is deepest in themselves.

Pierre Teilhard de Chardin

Sometimes, we find our greatest lessons when we must let go of something that has particularly brought us pleasure in the past. For example, Michael and I used to enjoy dancing. We were so good on the dance floor together! It was really our joy. But there came a time when I was unable to stand, much less dance.

We were at a party where there was dancing, and I nudged Michael and said, "Go ask Sheryl to dance." Now Sheryl is a great dancer. She is beautiful. She is wonderful. I had no idea how well she danced until that evening. I watched Michael and her glide and flow across the dance floor with the music, just and Michael and I used to do. And I can't say it wasn't unsettling for a moment. Then I looked at Michael's face and his expression of joy and his full-bodied movements as he threw himself into the dance. As I became more aware of his pleasure, I was able to share in this moment with him; my sense of loss vanished, replaced by a new kind of joy that I felt with him and through him.

One woman came up to me and remarked that if she were in my place, she'd kill Michael—*and* that woman dancing with him. She told me I had to be crazy to allow him to dance with her! I under-stood what she was saying, but when I love someone as much as I love Michael, I find great pleasure in that person's pleasure. I knew that I could no longer dance with him, and I found that there was something healing in allowing myself to enjoy his pleasure. The loss I felt—I wish it were me! It should be me! Why is this happening to me? Woe is me!—dissipated as I watched two people I love very much having a really wonderful time. This was the reality of the situation. This was the truth of the here and now. I couldn't be with him out there on the dance floor, so I had to enjoy the experience in a different way.

What I glimpsed at that moment was a connection to a greater spirit or source. This was the universal energy of love, wholeness, and connectedness. We glimpse it through love, through intuition, through collective memories, through dreams, personal visions— and through two people having a really wonderful time dancing.

It would have been easy for me to focus on potential negative aspects of the situation. After all, another woman dancing with my husband, as I had once been able to do, could easily become the source of jealousy and resentment and anger. But something had allowed me to see beyond this, to catch a glimpse of myself viewing life in a very different way, choosing pleasure instead of this darker alternative. I was literally led to an inner knowing that was healing in and of itself. I felt myself move closer to Spirit and to the freedom of truth.

As I confronted the fact that I had wrapped up my identity in things that I've physically done—the dancing, the drawing, dressing myself, or whatever—my previous investment in the physical *doing* began to melt away. And as it did, I discovered something beyond it. What I began to see was that my measure of worth did not need to be wrapped up in my actions or physical accomplishments. I saw that there clearly is a way that we participate in life that is quite beyond that. The breakthrough I experienced that evening was that, as we give up our physical identification, we discover the spiritual. And this seems to happen even for those who, like me, never thought of themselves as spiritual before.

Life Skill #3

Using your journal, record any stories or anecdotes you have heard, or firsthand experiences you have had, where a person (maybe you) transformed what initially appeared to be a very negative situation into a positive one. For models to get you started, think about some of the stories and anecdotes from this chapter—the ones about Sheryl, Matisse, and Renoir, for example.

LETTING GO IS TO RELAX; LETTING GOD IS TO BE PATIENT

Between us there is but a narrow wall
And by sheer chance, for it would take
Merely a call from your lips or mine to break it down,
And that without a sound.

Rainer Maria Rilke

There was no question that there was a loss in my not being able to dance with Michael, but once I acknowledged this reality, it was much easier to open up to the alternative pleasures that could be found. I did not have to get stuck with nothing more than my sense of loss. Rather, I could move on and take in different forms of pleasure that were available to me.

This was my first experience with what I would come to know as acceptance. At first, I was very doubtful that this kind of acceptance could lead to new openings, to new experiences that could be at least as fulfilling as those things I was giving up. I did not understand how it could really happen. But it did happen, and it would take me quite a while to fully grasp what had occurred and take advantage of all the doors this experience had opened up for me.

If it is true that living successfully with serious illnesses or injuries hinges on our ability to address our emotions and how we perceive our lives, where do we begin? What is the process that will carry us to the point when our greatest losses may allow us to look at life in a brand-new way, one in which we can find joy and a reason to celebrate our lives?

We begin by acknowledging to ourselves some of the more salient facts about our lives right now in the immediate present. You can record these by writing them down in a notebook for that purpose, recording them on a small tape recorder, or sharing them with a close friend or caregiver.

For example, like most others who have serious illnesses, I mourn the loss of simple pleasures such as physical comfort, which I once took so much for granted.

I feel the pain that comes when I don't stretch my legs often enough. I feel the bottoms of my feet in constant tremor, especially in the early morning or in response to the humid Philadelphia weather.

I can no longer get around, even in my own house, without the aid of my electric scooter. The two of us are an inseparable team.

I am unable to walk barefoot on the beach, a small pleasure I once deeply enjoyed.

There are many places I can't go because there are no spaces for people who are handicapped in the parking lot.

Where I go is limited to places where there are no curbs to impede travel in my electric scooter. This leaves out many restaurants, banks, movie theaters, and shopping centers where I might otherwise go.

To get you started, here are some questions and exercises, adapted from *How to Survive the Loss of a Love*, by Melba Colgrove, Ph.D., Harold H. Bloomfield, M.D., and Peter McWilliams. In this book, the authors map out a path through the loss we suffer when a loved one has died or moved away, or has divorced you, or has left home for reasons such as going away to college, getting a job in another town, and so on. The same principles that apply to these losses apply to our situation as well.

The more the marble wastes, the more the statue grows.

Michelangelo

1. What loss or losses are you experiencing in your life right now? What have you lost?

SAMPLE ANSWER:
I always took pride in my handwriting. However, now I can only write with difficulty, and what I write is often illegible. For an artist, this loss was devastating.

2. What other, less obvious, or seemingly not so serious losses have you had to face as a result of your illness?

SAMPLE ANSWER:
I used to enjoy feeling the sand under my feet when I walked on the beach. Now I cannot walk on the beach, nor can I feel the sand, because I have only a little sensation in the soles of my feet.

As you consider each of your losses, it is important to let yourself experience any feelings that come up. In this part of the process, just try putting a label on the emotion or emotions you are feeling. Work with one experience of loss at a time. Here is a list of primary emotions that most people associate with various parts of their losses. Scan the list quickly and see which of these twenty-four emotions best apply to the situations you have described.

Numb	Silly	Giddy
Indecisive	Hurt	Angry
Relieved	Happy	Feeling inferior
Melancholy	Frightened	Feeling like a failure
Envious	In pain	Listless
Outraged	Suicidal	Exhausted
Self-Hating	Beaten	Joyous
Overwhelmed	Fearful	Disgusted

After you have begun to identify the areas where you feel loss, along with the emotions associated with that loss, you have gone as far as you need to go with this first step. Do not attempt to *figure anything out* at this point. When you go on to the next chapter, you'll be looking at the process of mourning the losses you are experiencing, but try not to get too far ahead of yourself with the process.

As you identify some of the losses you are experiencing, and the emotions associated with them, try to put them in the context of our discussions in this chapter. Begin looking at them not as absolute facts, not as being carved in granite, but as dynamic inner processes, perceptions that are open to change and reinterpretation.

The stars receive their brightness from
the surrounding dark.

Dante

2

What We Remember: Mourning Our Losses and Letting Go

It isn't for the moment you are stuck that you need courage, but for the long uphill climb back to sanity and faith and security.

Anne Morrow Lindberg

In modern life we receive very little support or guidance to help us deal with loss. The grieving process, whether it is around the loss of money, objects, friends, personal abilities, or life itself, mostly has negative connotations. If you are like most people who grew up in this society, you've probably encountered subtle and not so subtle cautions against all forms of grieving. Think of the popular slogans associated with expressing loss: "Big boys don't cry!" "Stop feeling sorry for yourself!" "You've got to keep a stiff upper lip!" "You've got to be strong!" "Don't be a crybaby!"

Because of this negative conditioning around expressing loss, we can hardly expect to escape the belief that it is something we should avoid, something taboo or shameful, a sign of weakness or self-pity. For many of us, there is a sense of mystery about the meaning of loss and grief. They slip through the back door like a thief, sneaking into our lives uninvited, and often with many contradictory feelings surrounding them. And they can be a dark mystery! There can even be the sense that should we enter this mysterious or forbidden emotional territory we will drown in an ocean of sadness, tears, and grief. We've all heard people say they were afraid that if they ever started thinking about a loss they had suffered, they'd start crying and never stop. However, if you are truly familiar with this territory, if you have faced your grief, allowed yourself to feel it, and have cried over it, you know mourning is above all else a liberation, a way of freeing yourselves from the inner prison of your own deep depression, disappointment, anger, bitterness, fear, resentment, longing, guilt, and blame.

MAYBE WE ARE MORE THAN OUR EMOTIONS

Grief teaches the steadiest minds to waver.

Sophocles

The first thing to understand about grief and mourning is that it takes far more energy to push them away or hold them back than it takes to meet them head on and allow ourselves to feel these emotions. The energy we invest in holding back represents an important personal resource that we could best use in other ways. It is literally the energy of the life force within us, a force that we must learn to direct toward our own healing, whether that healing is physical, mental, emotional, spiritual, or all four simultaneously.

It can be helpful to think of our denial of loss and grief as being like a dam built across a wild river. The longer we hold it in place, the higher the water level rises and the greater the pressure against the dam becomes. And so we build the dam ever higher and stronger, reinforcing it against the accumulating pressure, while below the dam, along the riverside that represents the future, the land grows dry and parched.

The ability to mourn opens up the wild river that our lives really are, the vibrant, ever-changing flow of energy that carries us forward, that excites us with discovery of new things, new ways of seeing, new relationships. To find that this wild river could once again open up to me, in spite of the disease that daily robbed me of activities I'd once loved, was not only a great revelation but, in time, also a great source of joy.

I am aware, of course, that when we are struggling with the harsher realities of a serious illness, learning to mourn our losses may not appear to be a very high priority. But the fact is that if you are to live successfully with your illness, it may be one of the most important things you can do for yourself.

LEARNING TO LET GO

Suffering is a revelation. One discovers things one never discovered before.

Oscar Wilde

Above all, mourning is *letting go*. But letting go of what? Previously, you'll recall, we spoke of the role perception plays in our lives, that we can literally be imprisoned by clinging to what we think life "ought" to be, instead of living according to *what is* right now, in this moment. The long list of feelings we experience around loss comes from holding on to our perceptions about the way things "ought to be." When we are able to let go of these perceptions, it is as if we open a door to a brand-new world of possibility. To use an earlier metaphor, mourning our losses is a way to take apart the dam (our past perceptions of what life "should be") and let the river flow. When we do this, life reaches out to us in ways that we may never have even imagined before. Free of our perceptions of how life "ought to be," we provide ourselves with an opportunity to find another way of looking at the world. This is the source of genuine healing for all of us, able-bodied or not, a freedom from the illusions of life and an opening to the deeper meanings of our lives.

FOUR FOCAL POINTS FOR CHANGE

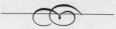

*The strangest and most fantastic fact about negative
emotions is that people actually worship them.*

P. D. Ouspensky

As we go forward with this chapter, keep the following four points
in mind:

1. At first, nearly everyone who has grown up in this society has
negative associations with mourning and letting go. Remember,
however, that prejudices against expressing the feelings of loss are
just that—*prejudices*. One of the biggest challenges we face with
learning to mourn and let go has to do with changing that prejudice
in our own minds. Of course, that change is itself a letting go.

2. While it may appear that our lives are determined by forces
outside us, over which we can never hope to have any control, we
can free ourselves of these forces by looking at our own perceptions,
mourning our losses, and letting go. We then open up to life's new
opportunities and directions. Even when it appears that we have no
choices, we must be careful not to shut down and close ourselves off
from other people (and ourselves); when we do, we are closing
ourselves off from choices presented to us at every moment.

3. The energy we put into denying and holding back feelings that
we may consider negative or scary is a valuable personal resource
that we can release and use for healing, ultimately embracing a new
"quality of life."

4. Though it may at first seem like we are doing just the opposite,
mourning and letting go of our perceptions about how we think life
should be is a way to totally embrace our lives—perhaps for the first
time.

IT'S REALLY OKAY TO FEEL DEPRESSED*

*The longer we dwell on our misfortunes, the greater is
their power to harm us.*

Voltaire

One of the earliest reactions we have to loss is depression. Biologists even tell us that this response is built into the system; at times of great grief or fear, the human organism and most other animals react in one of three ways—by fighting, by running away, or by numbing ourselves. Depression is the way most humans express the latter. When we are faced with a life-threatening illness, or one that involves the loss of abilities and functions we once considered necessary parts of our lives, we might try to fight or run, too, but because of the nature of these threats there are going to be times when we just fold up and withdraw into ourselves.

In many cases, depression is a normal and healthy response to an extremely challenging situation. However, there is no denying that it can also be both uncomfortable and frightening. We may barely be able to function, just dragging ourselves through the day. When we're in the middle of it, life becomes quite bleak, indeed. We tend to push people away, and this pushing away can be very disconcerting to those who care for us. There is no denying that it challenges us both in our individual lives and in our relationships to those around us. But there is also no denying that it is a normal response for most people faced with a serious illness.

---

*Is there no pity sitting in the clouds,
That sees into the bottom of my grief?*

William Shakespeare

---

* If you feel you are clinically depressed, by all means discuss this with your doctor or therapist. How can you tell if you are clinically depressed? Clinical depression is marked by a sense of utter hopelessness, wondering if life is worth living. Some people feel it is like a chemical reaction taking over their bodies. The depression I'm describing in this section of the book is more run-of-the-mill depression, what most people call the blues, the blahs, the sort of feeling most people refer to when they say with a sigh, "I'm depressed!"

What is the best way through depression? The way through always begins by acknowledging our dark feelings, not by denying them. At this time, it can also help to think of this acknowledgment as a first step down a path that will ultimately lead us to a place of peace and power, where we can again feel that our lives are worthwhile and meaningful.

One of the words often used to describe depression is *dissociation*. When we are in this state we barely function, able to put out only minimal energy to participate in life. Some people describe the feeling in nearly mystical terms: "as if I've just left my body"; "as if I'm anesthetized." More common is the feeling that "My whole body feels like it's made out of lead." Along with this experience, often described as withdrawal, there is sometimes confusion, an inability to make the simplest decisions or requests. This is the state of "I just want the world to go away" when we're being confronted with a sense of loss.

Usually, the loss being experienced is identified with a particular area of the body. For that reason, it can be extremely helpful to open your personal journal and *draw a simple outline of your body on a piece of paper* and either *circle or color in the area or areas where you are feeling the loss.* You may be surprised to discover the outcome of this exercise. Many people find that a sense of loss that is associated with a specific organ or limb may also involve other body areas, the obvious ones being the heart or head. In this respect, our impressions of loss can be quite individualized and subjective. The main purpose of this drawing exercise is to give our sense of loss a physical location, or locations, to help *ground* or *center* us as we go forward with the letting go process.

If you would have me weep, you must
first of all feel grief yourself.

Horace

GIVE IT A NAME

Once you've identified the areas associated with your sense of loss, go on to explore some of the ways you might describe the depression you're feeling. Here's a checklist that you may find helpful. If you wish, check off the symptoms that best apply to you.

- Regret
- Feeling left out or overlooked
- Exploding in rage or irritability over seemingly small things
- Indifference
- Lacking meaning or purpose
- Suffering head, neck, back, stomach, or other aches
- Withdrawn, isolated
- Restlessness
- Overeating or loss of appetite
- Feeling unappreciated or taken for granted
- Difficulty concentrating or remembering
- Pessimism
- Worrying and despair
- Fatigue and low energy
- Making errors
- Lacking confidence or motivation
- Rigidity or compulsiveness
- Agitation
- Outrage
- Sense of abandonment
- Feeling victimized

Understand that you do not have to *do* anything with these words or phrases other than to just be aware of them. Each step in this process simply brings you closer to the goal of coming to terms with your illness and reclaiming your life.

Life Skill #4

The easiest cure for the run-of-the-mill depression is movement—active, physical movement. Get up and do something. Stretch. Bend and touch your toes. Take a walk. Reach for something high over your head. Get your energy moving. It helps to do something that is even remotely productive. You'll get the physical boost of the movement and the psychological boost of the accomplishment. Don't wait until you "feel" you have enough energy to move out of the depression —start moving and the energy will be there. If you are confined to bed, or your movements are restricted, consult with your physician. Visualize and imagine yourself moving your body, singing and dancing, shifting from a stagnated focus to a vital, active approach. Talk to your physical therapist, if you have one. Ask about ways to stimulate the effects of movement through massage or physical therapy.

IT'S REALLY OKAY TO FEEL ANGER

If you would not have affliction visit you twice, listen at once to what it teaches.

James Burgh

Just as with depression, we're generally taught that it is suspicious, spiteful, jealous, indignant, malicious, and shameful to express anger. But my own experience with multiple sclerosis has taught me that our anger toward illness generally harbors a very positive expression of the life force itself. Once we get in touch with that anger, we are not far from embracing the healthy aspects these feelings represent.

Feeling anger when we learn of a serious illness is the most human reaction in the world. And recognizing that anger by getting in touch with the feeling and identifying what specifically is triggering it is part of the mourning process, one of the things we must do to let go. Feelings such as resentment and bitterness are closely associated with the kind of anger we're describing here. Ask yourself what you resent about being the person facing the loss. You'll find that completing the following sentences can help in this.

I'm furious about _____.

I hate it when _____.

I want to yell or scream whenever _____.

I'm disgusted by _____.

I'm fed up with _____.

I can't stand _____.

Each time we allow ourselves to feel, and then express our anger, we are letting go. The feelings we experience around our illness are not, as they say, "cast in concrete." Nor is there any great mystery about them. Each step we take to acknowledge and express them is one more step closer to letting go.

IT'S REALLY OKAY TO FEEL GUILT

*Perhaps someday it will be pleasant
to remember even this.*

Virgil

For many of us with serious illnesses, there is a sense of guilt, sometimes only vague but at other times quite powerful. The source of it may range from feeling that had we lived differently, or had we seen a doctor sooner, or had we only been more cautious in something we did, we would not have to be facing the difficulties and pain we are facing today. But guilt can take other forms as well. We may feel that we should have taken greater advantage of our good health when we were younger. Maybe there was something we had always dreamed of doing that we put off too long, and now can never hope to do. We may feel guilt about many situations closely or distantly associated with our illness.

To help you identify these areas, you might wish to try completing the following sentences:

If only_____.

I regret that_____.

I wish I had_____.

I wish I hadn't_____.

Maybe if I had_____.

Maybe if I hadn't_____.

I still feel guilty because_____.

I feel guilty that_____.

As an example of how guilt can work in our lives, let me draw from a recent experience of my own. This one has to do with regret and guilt I feel about not having a child earlier in my life. Not long ago, I was at a baby shower for my friend Laura, and felt a familiar tug of grief and guilt associated with having babies. It brought up an old sense of loss I hadn't realized was still there. "This is what good people do," a little voice said inside me. "They have babies. How can you claim to be a *good person* when you didn't do this? You thought only of your career and your art."

Intellectually, I knew that we all make choices and follow certain expectations and dreams we have for ourselves. Mine had indeed centered on my artwork and career, and most of the time I certainly had no regrets. But now, this old grievance crept in silently, whimpered, and made itself known. Before I could look at it and let it go, I had gone through the cycle of self-flagellation that so often accompanies guilt: pain, self-judgment, telling ourselves we are unworthy, pushing away pleasures and people's love or help because we feel we don't deserve them.

Applying the above list of phrases helped me identify the source and content of my guilt. Filling in the sentences in my journal, I wrote:

- *If only* I had decided to have a baby when I was twenty.
- *I regret that* I never even wanted to have a child until it was too late.
- *I regret that* my career was more important to me than becoming a mother.
- *I wish I had* thought this situation through a little bit more.
- *I wish I hadn't* been so insistent on not having a child, being so independent, etc.

It can, of course, be quite painful to go over these sources of guilt. But do so knowing that the process will bring you closer to that time when you will no longer be haunted by these feelings. Remember that even as we push these feelings back, pressing them as well as we can from our minds, they are there in the background, casting gray shadows over everything we do.

DO YOUR MOURNING NOW

Never does a man know the force that is in him till some mighty affection or grief has humanized the soul.

Frederick W. Robertson

The depression, anger, and guilt you feel are all products of your inner perception about the way you think life ought to have turned out for you. Keep in mind that as long as we hold on to these perceptions, the present will be colored by these feelings. To live successfully with your illness, you must release yourself from these old perceptions and turn your attention to what is. It is only in the present—regardless of what that present holds for us—that we can experience the ecstasy of life. This is what living successfully with illness is all about.

As we get in touch with these feelings, we give ourselves time to cry, to grieve over the perception of our life that we are letting go. Some people prefer to grieve alone, shutting off the phone and putting a DO NOT DISTURB sign on the door. Others prefer to find another person, who is compassionate, understanding, and would feel privileged to be with you through this time.

There are many ways to focus your attention on the perceptions from which these feelings come. Here are a few suggestions:

- Look at mementos, photos, or any other reminders of what you perceive you have lost.
- Rent a movie or watch TV shows that are likely to make you cry over losses similar to your own.
- Play music that evokes your sadness.
- Recall active happy times with friends or loved ones, prior to your illness.

We know too much and feel too little.

Bertrand Russell

As you draw closer and closer to your feelings of loss, and get more in touch with the perceptions of life that trigger them, start verbalizing what is occurring for you. To do this, try completing the following sentences:

I mourn because_____.

I feel sad because_____.

I can't accept_____.

I cry about_____.

I wish_____.

I can't believe that_____.

I grieve for_____.

This February, during the broadcast of the Winter Olympics women's figure skating competition, the graceful skaters reminded me of my former athletic self. Feeling heavyhearted, I used the above format to identify what was going on with me so that I wouldn't get stuck in my sense of loss. I embraced my grief and melancholy, holding myself close. I felt envious. My eyes welled up with tears again. I grieved for my loss, yet, realized that on the path my life has taken, I too have come to appreciate commitment to excellence and the tremendous endurance it takes to follow a dream. I, too, have learned to present and experience a graceful image of dignity and courage. In opening up deeper to my grief, I began to experience a new, healthier perception of life, based on my present reality. By observing all that is happening inside me without attachment to end results—without judgment, without expectations or pressure on myself, without comparison to the women figure skaters or to my own athletic past—I feel freer to appreciate myself, not only for what I can do but for the divine essence of who I am.

In the past when watching the Olympics, I felt crippled. Today, I feel like a beloved child, free from the need to compare my life to these others. This process of healing is ongoing. There is an old saying, "That which doesn't destroy us makes us stronger." Life-threatening illness can be a strengthener, not necessarily to the body—but certainly to the character and to the spirit.

Life Skill #5

The important thing is not getting rid of guilt, anger, depression, grief, resentment as quickly as possible; the important thing is learning about yourself.

I'm still really vulnerable, and I am not denying that. Sometimes, I feel "it should be different," or "this is how my life was supposed to turn out." But at these times I remind myself to embrace my fears and the depression and include the pain as part of my ongoing healing process.

The pain, then, is part of the happiness. "That's the deal," says Joy Gresham to her husband, the author and Christian theologian C. S. Lewis, about her fatal illness in the 1994 film *Shadowlands*. Based on a true story, the film explores spirituality, the meaning of suffering, the pain of loss, and an understanding that God helps people find their true path by occasionally making them suffer.

As you open up to your own grief, it may stir up memories of other losses that may or may not seem to have anything to do with your illness.

As farfetched as it may seem that these could be related to what's happening now, don't ignore these memories. Make note of them in your journal. For example, you might have lost a loved one during your childhood or adolescence, and the memory comes up now. Or perhaps there was a business loss in your early adult life that still haunts you. Let these come alive in your memory. And then allow them to pass through, letting go of them along with the other perceptions you have held on to in your mind.

This cup holds grief
and balm
in equal measure. Light, darkness.
Who drinks from it must change.

May Sarton

As we recall losses, get in touch with anger, and feel the heaviness of our depression, fears may arise. Let yourself feel these fears. Don't attempt to push them away at this time. Feel them, then articulate them, preferably in writing or in the presence of another person. To do this, you might wish to fill in the following sentences:

I fear_____.

I am afraid that_____.

I am terrified of_____.

I feel scared about_____.

If a door slams shut it means that God is pointing to an
open door further on down.

Anna Delaney Peale

Letting Go of Our Addictions to Negative Thinking

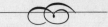

*We are born believing. A man bears beliefs
as a tree bears apples.*

Ralph Waldo Emerson

In recent years, millions of people throughout the world have healed their lives through the twelve-step programs. While you might wonder what this could possibly have to do with healing our perceptions about illness, there are those who believe that twelve-step processes work precisely because they address and alter our perceptions about the way life ought to be.

Take a few minutes to read through the Twelve Steps, substituting the words *negative thinking* whenever you see the word *alcohol* or *alcoholics*. While you may not want to follow all of them just now, pick out one or two that catch your attention or that you feel you might be willing to explore.

A Healing Prayer for This Time

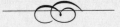

THE TWELVE STEPS

1. We admitted we were powerless over alcohol [or other substances or behaviors] and that our lives had become unmanageable.

2. Came to believe that a Power greater than ourselves could restore us to sanity.

3. Made a decision to turn our will and our lives over to the care of God as we understood Him.

4. Made a searching and fearless moral inventory of ourselves.

5. Admitted to God, to ourselves, and to another human being the exact nature of our wrongs.

6. Were entirely ready to have God remove all these defects of character.

7. Humbly asked Him to remove our shortcomings.

8. Made a list of all persons we had harmed, and became willing to make amends to them all.

9. Made direct amends to such people wherever possible, except when to do so would injure them or others.

10. Continued to take personal inventory and when we were wrong promptly admitted it.

11. Sought through prayer and meditation to improve our conscious contact with God as we understood Him, praying only for knowledge of His will for us and the power to carry that out.

12. Having had a spiritual awakening as a result of these steps, we tried to carry this message to alcoholics, and to practice these principles in all our affairs.

In his book *Magnificent Addiction*, Philip Kavanaugh, M.D., states that "Addiction to our beliefs . . . is at the core of all addictions." In this case, we might substitute the word *perceptions* for *beliefs.* To hold on to our beliefs of how life *ought to be,* instead of embracing *what is,* we truly are like addicts clinging to the behavior or addictive substance that cripples us.

Dr. Kavanaugh and many other therapists who have experienced both addiction and healing in their own lives, state that there is a core addiction—the addiction to control. The alcoholic has the illusion that his use of alcohol gives him control over his life— when, of course, just the opposite is true. And we all, to one degree or another, use our perceptions of the way life ought to be as an illusion of control—that is, we believe that as long as we hold on to our perceptions, we have control over our lives. There is, of course, a certain amount of truth in this. However, clinging to perceptions that are clearly no longer applicable is easily as destructive as the alcoholic's clinging to his perception that alcohol gives him control over his life.

Admitting that our perceptions no longer serve us, or that the illusion of control we once found in our addiction not only doesn't work for us but is making our lives miserable, is a key step in every twelve-step program. In fact, it is a key ingredient in every process of personal change, stated or not.

When a man is willing and eager, the gods join in.

Aeschylus

Dr. Kavanaugh teaches that we never give up our addictions (perceptions); rather, we upgrade them. He believes that to live successfully, we must understand that our perceptions are nothing more or less than they really are—a system of beliefs and feelings that we have chosen to guide our lives. Because we have chosen them, we have the power to change and improve them. This is how we grow, and this is how we learn to live successfully with our illness.

An important part of the twelve-step process is to take one step at a time—to do what you can do right now. Be respectful of the fact that we grow gradually and we expand in our abilities with each step we take.

Those who are familiar with twelve-step programs may be familiar with the "Serenity Prayer," which addresses the issue of control and letting go very well. Many have found this prayer invaluable when in the process of letting go and mourning past perceptions:

> God grant me the Serenity
> To accept the things I cannot change,
> The courage to change the things I can,
> And the wisdom to know the difference.

You do not have to be religious to benefit from prayers of this kind. I have learned that even people who are antireligious or who consider themselves to be agnostics find that prayers at this time help them let go. One cannot help but be reminded of powers greater than ourselves, that in letting go we literally create a possibility for a new view of the world, and our lives, to come in. One of the simplest reminders for this is contained in a meditation that appears in many different forms in many different spiritual disciplines.

Let go. Let God.

Letting go means to relax and be patient. Letting God means being open and accepting whatever the Spirit brings to us. Letting go is something we must choose to do; it is an ongoing process that takes place in one day or in one moment. As we go forward, mourning the past perceptions that have served us, and letting go, each new day brings new opportunities and offers new directions. We see these opportunities only if we remain awake and responsive in the present, no longer trying to force the realities of today into the old perceptions of how life should be.

IT TAKES GREAT STRENGTH
TO REACH FOR GOD

Yea, though I walk through the valley of the shadow of death, I will fear no evil: for thou art with me; thy rod and thy staff they comfort me.

Psalm 23

It can appear, at times, that we have no choices or that our choices are extremely limited. But in spite of what appears to be, we must be careful not to shut down, not to close off our feelings from ourselves and other people. When we do shut down, we also close ourselves off to the new directions presented to us. Shutting down, trying not to feel the pain, is a common reaction in mourning our losses. Yet, in the long run, we make our lives much more difficult and painful for ourselves when we choose to go numb—perhaps the most common way we humans have for coping with difficult situations. In this numbed state, we can't possibly go forward. The fact is that we feel increasingly separate from other people and from life itself. As contradictory as it might seem, the only way to open up to life is to stand tall and walk through the pain.

Life Skill #6

*C*hange the image. This exercise activates a "warning light" that reminds us to *change the image or the action*—before taking part in the contrary action. Ask yourself what you are upset about, and accept whatever it is. Give yourself permission to do what you or they *have already done*. Allow your image of yourself to adjust to the reality of being a human being.

What's the payoff? Ask yourself what you are getting from this. More guilt? Feeling better?

Breathe. Anger, depression, resentment, and guilt are usually felt in the stomach, abdomen, shoulders, jaw, or chest. Take slow, deep breaths into these areas as you breathe in. Imagine a white light going in with each breath and filling the area as you sacrifice your guilt. Just give it up.

As you work with your old perceptions, letting go through mourning your losses, pray for the support to recognize that there truly is nothing to be gained by holding on. Things have changed. The truth of the matter is that what you're trying to hold on to doesn't even exist anymore. Letting go is ultimately the work of the heart much more than the mind. It isn't enough to go through the motions of letting go. We have to sincerely be willing to sacrifice our loss and despair so that we are able to move forward with our lives into *what is* our present reality rather than clinging desperately to what is now in the past.

THE ILLNESS / 71

SELF NURTURING, AN ESSENTIAL INGREDIENT

*The most beautiful music of all is the music
of what happens.*

Old Irish tale

The process of mourning and letting go takes a tremendous amount of energy. Think of this as a time of healing, of old wounds closing up, of your body, mind, and spirit coming together as a whole. Just as with a physical injury, your body and mind possess powerful self-healing capacities that do not function in a vacuum. Your conscious cooperation with these innate abilities is important at this time. Here are some suggestions for ways you can do this.

Rest whenever possible. Everyone knows the healing powers of sleep, but not all of us give ourselves the permission to rest when we are in crisis. There is a tendency to think that we have to stay busy, to be always *doing*. Remind yourself that rest is, in the long run, productive and therapeutic.

Learn to meditate. Meditation is the perfect model for letting go. It is literally a way to quiet our minds, to slow down or stop that part of the brain and nervous system that is responsible for perception.

If you are not already in the habit of meditating, you can learn the process, which is really quite simple. There is a variety of meditation tapes available in most bookstores.

Spend time quietly in nature. Most of us find nature both inspiring and healing. When we are out on a favorite beach or walking in a quiet woods, there is a sense of peace and harmony that comes. There is a way in which the harmony that we find there helps us feel more at peace within ourselves. It is in this peaceful place that the healing capacities of body and mind are at their best. The pleasure we find in a simple excursion in nature can truly be beneficial in every way.

Take a hot bath. For centuries, warm water has been employed for its therapeutic effects. Soothing heat relaxes tense muscles and helps to open capillaries, carrying healing nutrients to organs throughout our bodies. When you cannot take baths, soak your feet for similar therapeutic benefits. (Remember to consult with your physician if you are sensitive to heat and humidity, or if you have an immuno-logical condition which could be aggravated by hot baths.)

Listen to restful music. Like meditation, soothing music helps us let go of perceptions that no longer serve us well. For some sugges-tions, refer to "For Further Listening" in the resources section (page 225).

Talk to plants. If you are a plant person, you may find solace and a special kind of comfort in talking to your plants. It appears to offer the same comforts as spending time in nature.

Talk to pets. In most ancient cultures, animals were seen as media-tors between people and the powers of nature. It was believed that even though animals did not possess the gift of language, they helped remind humans of their spiritual identity. Perhaps our pets serve a similar function, reminding us of the power of unconditional love. My cats are wonderful teachers.

Pray. I engage in some sort of daily spiritual practice. This is my private time between myself and God. Whether you are religious or not, set aside time to just be quiet. Listen and be open to support that comes from within. The spiritual life is our inner life, and anyone who is learning how to live successfully with illness will find both comfort and guidance through a connection to the God within them. Daily spiritual practice builds a meaningful inner life. Your prayer might be like this: How can I awaken, expand, enhance, heighten, or magnify my experience of a Spirit greater than myself?

---

*Certain thoughts are prayers. There are certain moments
when, whatever be the attitude of the body,
the soul is on its knees.*

Victor Hugo

KEEP DECISIONS TO A MINIMUM

One ought every day at least to hear a little song, read a good poem, see a fine picture, and, if it were possible, to speak a few reasonable words.

Johann Wolfgang von Goethe

When you are going through the process of mourning and letting go, a lot is happening inside you. From the outside it can appear that very little is going on, but this is hardly the case. If you are truly letting go of old perceptions, and allowing new perceptions to form, you are changing—and quite possibly changing in some rather significant ways. For this reason, it is important to put off as many decisions as possible. Remember, the nature of change is that in a month, six months, or even a year, you literally are not going to be holding the same beliefs you hold today. Different things will be important to you. You'll have different priorities.

Make a list of at least six decisions you will *not* be making for at least a month. Actually write them down. And also record a date, one month from today, when you will consider this issue again. If you worry about any of the things on your list before the date you've recorded, tell yourself, "It's okay. I'll make that decision after such-and-such a date." You will find there are very few things in the world that require immediate decisions. For now, the more you can put off, the better.

WHAT COMFORTS YOU?

Experience everybody (or everything) in your life as either a teacher or a lover.

Ken Keyes, Jr.

It is important to take good care of yourself in a very special way during this time. For many people, this isn't easy to do. Remember, this is a time when you may be struggling with feelings of unworthiness. Though these feelings will pass as you go through the mourning process, you may find that it isn't easy to give yourself permission to treat yourself well.

What exactly does it mean to take care of yourself? It means being able to experience the feelings of being cared for and nurtured. Above all, it means *loving yourself*. Here are just a few suggestions for ways to do that:

Get a massage. This could be from a close friend or from a professional massage therapist. Some people prefer full body massage, while others feel tremendously nurtured by a good foot or neck massage. We know that in terms of the body's own self-healing mechanisms that therapeutic massage has many potential benefits —physical, emotional, and spiritual.

Get yourself a special treat. This could be flowers, chocolates, an article of clothing, or tickets to a concert.

Do something special with a friend or family member. This could include going out to dinner or to a show, going shopping, going on a trip together, or spending a quiet evening at home.

Watch a favorite movie. Thanks to modern technology, it is now easy to get copies of favorite movies to watch in the privacy and comfort of home. To be entertained in this way, immersed in your favorite dramas, comedies, or musicals, is therapeutic in itself.

Get a hug or give a hug. In her lectures to audiences all over the country, Marianne Williamson frequently points out that "giving and receiving are the same." When we truly give to others, with no strings attached, we are nurtured in a wonderful way. This is especially true when it comes to good hugs.

Practice laying on of hands. Put your hands over your heart and feel the healing energy flow from your hands into your heart. Take a few moments whenever you feel the need to give yourself this special "healing."

Surround yourself with life. To be always in communion with life is wonderfully healing in itself. When faced with a serious illness, many people find comfort in a pet or having flowers delivered or growing beautiful plants around them. Visit a zoo. Start a garden. If you have a friend or relative with a new baby, invite them to visit. Go to live plays, concerts, dance performances, sporting events.

THE ILLNESS / 75

Cuddle with a teddy bear. When we were children, many of us had a favorite doll or stuffed toy, often a teddy bear, to which we clung when we were distressed. While it is a mystery why it works, thousands of people, children and adults, find comfort in this way. If you had such a *friend* when you were little, you might want to go to a toy store and find a similar toy that will comfort you now. I have a friend who sends beautiful, handmade teddy bears to loved ones she hears are going through difficult times. The thank-you letters she gets back frequently say what good "medicine" they are. My teddy bear's name is Sid. The telephone number for the Vermont Teddy Bear Co. is in the resources section (see page 245).

Be gentle with yourself. Sit down and make a list of the things you say to yourself or think about yourself that are harsh or critical. Then turn them around and make a list of the ways you can be kind, nurturing, and gentle to yourself. Be aware of your "self-talk" —that is, what we tell ourselves about ourselves. For most of us, a large amount of this self-talk is the voice of our own "inner critic," telling us what we do wrong but rarely patting us on the back or encouraging us. So make a point of consciously developing self-talk that is nurturing, loving, and encouraging. You will be surprised at how powerful this can be.

Give yourself permission to heal your loss at your own pace. So often, when we are faced with loss, we feel pressure to get over it as quickly as possible. Think of phrases like "stop feeling sorry for yourself and move on," which we hear so often in our society. While many of us can't just drop everything we're doing to mourn our losses, it is important not to cut the process short, either. Do what you must do but leave yourself time to mourn, even if it is just for a few moments at the end of the day. I often suggest to people that they write down ten good reasons to give themselves permission to heal their loss at their own pace.

We are healed of a suffering only by experiencing it to the full.

Marcel Proust

Seek external support. There can be great comfort in finding others like yourself, people who are going through the same challenges you are. This might mean joining a support group through a hospital or clinic you are familiar with or contacting social service agencies listed in your phone book to track down groups that offer camaraderie and the safe, familiar feeling that "we are in this together."

Life Skill #7

*A*ltitude is our viewing point, the perspective we have. The higher our viewing point, the more we can see. The more we can see, the more information we have. The more information we have, the better we can make well-informed decisions.

Attitude is the way we approach things. Look at this journey as an adventure to be enjoyed. The choice is yours. The key is your attitude.

The connection between altitude and attitude is easy to see. You can add upward momentum by raising your attitude. If we have a good attitude, our altitude will lift; if we have an elevated altitude, our attitude will rise.

Altitude is raised through meditation, prayer, spiritual practices, creativity, and service.

Attitude is lifted through inspiring lectures, reading, seminars, movies, support groups, television shows—concepts and techniques that naturally lead to an enlightened approach to learning.

Try it. They work in harmony with each other.

WORDS OF SELF-EMPOWERMENT AND ENCOURAGEMENT

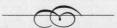

You gain strength, courage, and confidence by every experience in which you really stop to look fear in the

face. You are able to say to yourself, "I lived through this horror. I can take the next thing that comes along."

Eleanor Roosevelt

As you move along through this letting go process, take time out to give yourself progress reports. Otherwise, we don't give ourselves credit for what we've accomplished. Look for new information that may have bubbled up along the way—areas that you had denied or pretended were "all better" but which you eventually looked at, grieved, and let go. Be sure to give yourself positive feedback for these achievements in your self-talk. In the beginning, you may not have wanted to do anything for other people, either, because you yourself felt wounded and deprived or because you did not feel that you had anything worthwhile to give. Note any changes in your desire to do more for others.

In your journal, you might want to write something about dealing with loss and what you have learned about yourself.

If you are of an artistic bent, draw a picture to express in a visual way some of the challenges you've been through. Draw a picture of how your inner strength feels or looks to you. Draw something about what it means to you to grow through your loss.

Now that you have become more familiar with this process of mourning and letting go, you may have your own prescriptions for self-healing. You might, for example, want to write a prayer or meditation tailored to what you now know about yourself and your own needs. See yourself as your own "physician of the soul," and administer to yourself wisely.

With a sharp eye on where you are now, imagine yourself living successfully with your illness, whole and healthy in the ways we have been exploring together in this book.

LET GO AND MOVE ON

As you draw to the end of this chapter, focus your attention on qualities in yourself that you most like and admire. They may be different from the ones you noted at the end of the last chapter or they may be the same. The point is to focus on yourself in a positive, nurturing way for a moment, reminding yourself that everything you have been reading and doing in this chapter has been aimed at helping you to live successfully with your illness.

Always be ready to remind yourself that healing is a process, not a single event. As on a long train ride, the journey is most enriching and enjoyable when we learn to relax and watch the scenery, leaving the "driving" to God.

Everyone's life is a fairy tale, written by God's fingers.

Hans Christian Andersen

3

What We Believe: Changing Our View of Illness

The more beliefs and conclusions you have about life, the less you are willing to explore the infinite wealth and beauty of life.

Gurudev (Yogi Amrit Desai)

No matter who you are, you grow up with certain myths and prejudices about what it means to have a serious illness and what it means to be labeled "handicapped." We have only to look at the language applied to us to have an insight into these prejudices. For example, consider the term *invalid*. Although pressure groups have helped to change the media's use of this term, it still lingers in the public consciousness, carrying the implication that when people have a serious illness or physical limitations they are somehow *not valid* as human beings.

Lobby groups over the past three decades have done much to

change public opinion about people who are physically challenged. They have made it possible for those of us in wheelchairs to become much more fully integrated with mainstream society, through providing special parking places, ramps, water fountains, elevators, and rest room facilities in public places and at work sites. While it can be argued that most communities have barely scratched the surface in this regard, the efforts made are helping to change everyone's perceptions about the actual capacities of people who are handicapped. Our beliefs about what it means to have a serious illness or a physical challenge are changing.

When most of us are first diagnosed or we wake up in a hospital one day to discover that our lives have been changed forever by an accident, all our worst fears and prejudices about what it means to be "handicapped" come crashing down around us. For a while, we may very well see ourselves as helpless victims, doomed to live as shadows of our former selves. We may get angry or deny what is happening to us. But whatever our reaction, we are certain to bump up against our own beliefs about what it means to be ill. Most people are very surprised by this, because until now those perceptions of what it means to be physically challenged had seemed to apply to other people. Even attitudes that once seemed benevolent toward people who are handicapped—for example, pity—can have serious ramifications when we find ourselves on the receiving end. We suddenly discover that being pitied can make us feel invisible or unworthy—not the equal of the person doing the pitying.

You have no idea what a poor opinion I have of myself—
and how little I deserve it.

W. S. Gilbert

There are very few people who have anything approaching a positive perception toward illness or physical limitation. Most of the time, our beliefs about illness make us feel pretty hopeless. In addition to that, more general perceptions, such as our self-judgments and negative reactions to our thoughts and habit patterns, are going to become a part of the mix, becoming hurdles we must surmount if we are to live successfully with our illness. The bottom line is that if we want to learn how to live with the *reality of what is present today*, regardless of our diagnosis or prognosis, we need to look as closely at these beliefs as we do at the physical condition itself. This begins by dissecting the anatomy of a belief—the heart of which is found in what consciousness researchers call "perception and projection."

A Short Course on Perception and Projection

Most of the time we think we're sick, it's all in the mind.

Thomas Wolfe

Like racial prejudice, our perceptions about what it means to be physically challenged are filled with beliefs and interpretations that begin in our own minds. If you understand how this works it's a lot easier to move beyond any self-limiting illusions and judgments you might have, and to go forward to live successfully with your illness or handicap.

For a moment, think of your mind as being something like a motion picture production studio. Every moment of our lives we are filming our experiences; we are recording in our minds volumes and volumes of images, conversations, thoughts, and feelings. It is from this huge library of experiences that we interpret or "make sense" of new opportunities and situations as they come into our lives. In fact, we make sense of the world largely by projecting our own films or memories outside us and onto other people and situations. It is as if our minds find a close match between the outside world and the films we have stored in our archives; then we project our own images onto that external situation. While this process is the source of many conflicts and misunderstandings in our lives, it also gives us some place to start.

Because our perceptions and projections rarely provide us with anything but a rough set of guidelines for responding to new situations, we have our greatest range of choices when we don't insist that what we perceive "out there" is our only alternative. These guiding perceptions only tell us what we have previously experienced in similar situations. They are like maps we've drawn up after traveling to places that were somewhat like this new territory we've entered—but only somewhat like them.

GUIDEPOSTS TO MASTERY

Always bear in mind that our own resolution to success is more important than any other one thing.

Abraham Lincoln

Our first reactions to new situations are predominantly projections of our perceptions and beliefs. But then, as we live day to day with that new situation, we begin to see that our projections don't exactly match up with the new reality. At the point when we recognize this, we have a choice: we can either insist on clinging to our projection—which is accurate only in terms of our own inner archives—or we can start looking more carefully at what's out there. Most of our lives, we go back and forth between these two points, trusting our projections part of the time, then opening up a little bit at a time to the external world.

To successfully negotiate any big changes in our lives, we must go through a process of first trusting our projections. As we see that they don't completely match the new way of life we've stepped into, we must slowly let go of our old projections and allow ourselves to experience the new reality. It's never an easy process, even when the new reality is something we've always wanted—such as getting married, moving to a new place, getting a new job, or buying a new car.

Never forget that within our own minds, back there in the archives where we have stored all our films, we have integrated not only social prejudices about being handicapped but also self-limiting beliefs fostered by our individual experiences of illness when we were children. All of these beliefs will have an impact on us in the here-and-now because, count on it, we will project them into our lives. The good news is that we need not be prisoners of our own perceptions and projections. Once we are able to identify them, we are well on our way toward making new choices about how we will live our lives. When we know the power of our projections, we can go in, edit our films, and create award-winning, five-star movies that will serve us better.

In this chapter we're going to be exploring some of these projections and irrational beliefs with the goal of identifying a course of action we might take to liberate ourselves from unnecessary limits we might place on ourselves. For many of us, the images we are dealing with begin with our memories of childhood illnesses.

Attachment is the great fabricator of illusions; reality can be attained only by someone who is detached.

Simone Weil

CHILDHOOD EXPERIENCES WITH ILLNESS

All of us collect fortunes when we are children—a fortune of colors, of lights and darkness, of movements, of tensions. Some of us have the fantastic chance to go back to our fortune when we grow up.

Ingmar Bergman

Most of us had childhood illnesses that for a period of time changed our lives. Maybe it was measles, chicken pox, or a bad case of the flu. If you can recall these times in your life, you will probably discover that you didn't even think about what the doctor or your parents called it. What you probably focused on was that your life was changed by it—at least temporarily. Maybe you couldn't go out to play for a day or two. Maybe you could not spend time with a special friend. Maybe you felt so uncomfortable that you had to stay in bed for several days in a row. Maybe people were loving and caring toward you during this time, maybe not. In some families, periods associated with illness are tense and high-strung, filled with very confusing messages for a child.

It takes one a long time to become young.

Pablo Picasso

No matter how significant or insignificant these events might seem to you now, the fact remains that they helped to form the feelings toward your illness that you are experiencing today. These early events are integral parts of your projections. By gently exploring them, you will begin to get some insights about the projections you are having to deal with in your present situation. These projections will not tell the whole story, of course, but they will begin to uncover the first components of the process of change that you'll have to work through if you are to live successfully with your present situation.

Take some time to briefly relive your early childhood experiences with illness. Record your findings in your journal, if you wish. Most people find it helpful to begin by focusing on simple physical details, such as what the sickroom looked like, any medicines you may have taken, unpleasant symptoms, or the memory of something your illness prevented you from doing. Pay particular attention to any details you might remember about your relationships with other people. You might want to use a tape recorder for this exercise.

- How did you feel about being dependent on others?
- How did your parents respond to your illness? Did you have the sense that your relationship with them changed because of your illness? If so, how did it change? Were they more loving? Less loving? Did the way they related to you help you to feel stronger? Weaker?
- Did you experience any benefits from being ill, such as getting more attention or quality time with your parents?
- Were there negative reactions to you as a result of your illness, such as being made to feel you were a burden to others?
- What kind of self-talk—judgments, blame, and so on—did you engage in when others (a parent, a physician, another family member, and so on) told you about the illness you had and what it would mean in terms of changing your life? Did you feel frightened, bewildered, angry, hopeless, despairing, and so on?

- What effects, short- or long-term, did this experience have on your self-image—that is, your sense of worthiness or unworthiness? For example: "I am damaged goods," "I am not good enough," "I am a helpless victim," "I am unlovable," "God is punishing me for something I did or failed to do," "I will never be good enough now."

God gave burdens, also shoulders.

Yiddish proverb

- Take a look at how your early experience of illness affected your sense of having control of your life. Much of our sense of well-being is based on these early impressions. Did being ill trigger a sense of your life being out of control? Did it have any impact on your sense that you could plan or not plan for the future, or that your vulnerability in this area would get in the way of your dreams for the future?

- Do you recall discovering sources of inner strength at the time? Were you self-supporting or self-judging? In what specific ways was this manifest?

- Did any experiences you had with medical professionals, a parent, or other caregiver at the time of your illness cause you to feel that you were "not enough," or that you should be perfect? For example, in my own journal entries I have noted my reaction to something a doctor once said while he was taking blood from my arm. He remarked that I had "very thin spindly veins," and without looking directly at me, said to his assistant, "I think we're going to have a problem here." I immediately began to judge myself and be very critical of my own body. This was exaggerated in my mind because I also believed that I had to be "perfect." Having "spindly veins" definitely meant to me that my health was not perfect, and I judged myself harshly about that.

Have no fear of perfection—you'll never reach it.

Salvador Dalí

As you make these notes in your journal, let yourself free-associate; if other situations come to mind as you are writing or thinking about the questions above, just allow them to come. Write them down too. It is often these memories that float spontaneously into our minds that prove to be the most revealing, mirroring back to us very clear reflections of our judgmental perceptions.

Most people write in their journals over a period of days, weeks, or even months. Every time you sit down to read over what you've already recorded or to make a new entry, you'll probably have new insights. Use your journal for any related memories or negative judgments that might come up for you around the subject of injury, illness, or physical handicap.

As you go along, notice that your awareness grows each time you do any journal work, either reading your old entries or making new ones. It is this growing awareness that leads you to greater and greater freedom and sense of choice.

As you work with your entries, ask yourself how the experiences you are reading or recording affect how you think about, feel, and look at your illness right now. How are you projecting old pictures onto your present situation? For example, if you were isolated from others when you were ill as a child, does the expectation of being isolated again cause you to feel anxious or upset? Or, if you were given special treatment that made you feel good about yourself when you were ill as a child, are you currently feeling deprived because you are not getting that treatment now, as an adult?

Know what you want to do, hold the thought firmly, and do every day what should be done. And every sunset will see you that much nearer the goal.

Elbert Hubbard

Recognize that thinking what you are thinking right now and feeling what you are feeling right now about your present situation are projections. They come from inside you, based on past experience. Even when you are quite sure that what you are thinking or feeling is totally "justified" by your present circumstances, the fact remains that it is still a projection. You might note that even our top scientists, Nobel Prize winners, and eminent researchers say that their most celebrated observations and discoveries are still projections. We can usually find evidence in the external world that proves that our perceptions are "correct." We want to acknowledge this; but what is important is to recognize that what we think and feel is a product of our own minds. Thus we can choose to change our projections, and as our projections change so does our life experience.

Life Skill #8

As you go through the day, work with your insights and the memories you have brought to the surface. When confronted with a difficult day, when you get very discouraged or frightened, take the time to trace what you are feeling back to your own archive of experiences. Make yourself a promise that there is another way of looking at the world and you are determined to find it. Even though you are faced with very profound physical challenges, be reminded that how you handle the challenge of change itself can make the difference between getting stuck in a very limiting perspective and living successfully with your illness.

LABELS SCHLABELS!

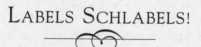

If you make friends with yourself, you will
never be alone.

Maxwell Maltz

Doctors are famous for labeling their patients. I am quite aware of having a long list of doctors and nurses in whose eyes I am not Linda Noble Topf but "the MS case with spindly veins." While it can have a devastating effect on you if you are the person with the illness, giving you the impression that in other people's minds you have become a disease and are no longer relevant as a person, one can see the other side of it—that these labels are useful within a doctor's system. Labels allow the medical professional to make a distinction between one set of symptoms and another. Also, when patients are appropriately labeled as having a recognized disease, the doctor, clinic, or insurance company is given assurance that the condition is "legitimate," thus justifying the treatment costs.

Never go to a doctor whose office plants have died.

Erma Bombeck

Pay attention to how these labels affect you. For most people labels are dehumanizing, to say the least. I am not Multiple Sclerosis. *Who I am is me.* And no matter how much time or expense or difficulty is involved with my having this illness, the fact remains that I am first and foremost me. I am not a set of symptoms in a medical book. I am not a list of treatment procedures on a medical bill. *I am me.*

In addition to having a negative impact in terms of self-esteem and a sense of worthiness, labels are restrictive in many other ways. If you have been labeled with an illness that the medical textbooks say is terminal, the medical system will tend to treat you that way even though there is abundant evidence that every day many people have spontaneous remissions, enjoying total recovery, or are discovered to not follow a typical pattern in the course of their illness. Like most things in life, diseases can have very individualized components; your influenza may involve the same virus, and have many of the same symptoms as mine, yet because our bodies, minds, and life experiences are different there can be nearly infinite variables. Furthermore, if we are labeled with a specific illness, the textbooks will prescribe a very specific course of treatment; most physicians don't believe in and will not try any treatment program that goes outside the officially sanctioned course of treatment. For them, it is as if no other possibility exists. However, when we study medical history—even over a ten-year-range—we discover that the diagnosis and treatment of most diseases change constantly, often quite dramatically, even reversing themselves.

Do or do not. There is no try.

Yoda

Labels can be limiting whether they are applied to illness or not: whether to engineer, invalid, doctor, housewife, victim, artist, butcher, baker, candlestick maker, lawyer, or Indian chief. We are always much more than our labels. Our concept of what any label means may be far removed from the human beings behind those labels. As John-Roger, an international educator, author, and friend, says, "When you get down to the essence, everyone is living love, and titles and other descriptions are irrelevant."

An Exercise to Help You Identify Labels

Great men are they who see that spiritual is stronger than any material force, that thoughts rule the world.

Ralph Waldo Emerson

This labeling exercise will help you identify some of the stereotypes and "automatic beliefs" you may be harboring about illness. Being able to capture the various negative labels that have become associated with your illness will be a powerful step toward your own greater freedom.

Read over the following list, with its stereotypes, your reactions to them, your resulting self-judgments, and the assumptions you've made about yourself. This list of stereotypes was drawn from my own personal experience, things I heard when I was growing up, or saw in movies or on television. Some are from encounters I've had with my family and with people I've worked with, from friends when they learned that I had MS, or from medical professionals. You may find that only a few things on this list strike a chord for you; you may find that they all do. And, of course, I would hope that you'd add your own experiences to this list.

As you go through this list, make note of any self-judgments you recognize. Jot down descriptions of these judgments and assumptions in your journal. Draw on your personal archives, memories, and self-talk. Remember that if you can intensify your awareness of negative labels and false assumptions, you can learn to make positive choices in how you perceive yourself.

STEREOTYPES	REACTIONS	SELF-JUDGMENTS	ASSUMPTIONS
Victim	Who, me?! (Hurt)	I'm not good enough.	With MS, I have to prove myself.
Crippled	Why me?! (Anger)	I am a bad person.	I'll never succeed.
Challenged	Not me!! (Denial)	I am being dependent.	I can't stand up for myself.
Disabled	Are you talking to me? (Disbelief)	I'm not attractive anymore. She's physically fit, therefore better than me.	He only sees my walk and my "problem"—not the real me.
Afflicted	You don't know me!! (I exist!)	I'm all alone in this.	She doesn't want the burden of being my friend.
Co-dependent	It's there.	He'll leave me.	I am powerless and helpless.
Dysfunctional	What makes you say that?	I'm a burden to him.	I have a reason to be!
Handicapped	Huh? I'm handicapable!	I can't do it myself.	I don't expect anything more from myself.
Sufferer	Nobody really knows!	I won't be able to compete.	It's in my upbringing!
Invalid	Feel sorry for me.	Only babies do this.	You will never leave.

IDENTIFYING NEGATIVE PERCEPTION

What we see depends mainly on what we look for.

John Lubbock

It is human nature to seek *justification* in the external world for the negative beliefs and perceptions that we hold in our mind. And, rest assured, the world is a big enough place that we can always find situations that would seem to prove our beliefs infallible. For example, we can argue, "Well, I don't go out to dinner because people in restaurants don't like to see people in wheelchairs." Or, "Nobody is going to hire me if they know about my epilepsy." Certainly, if we go out to dinner at enough large restaurants we are going to find people who don't like to see wheelchairs. And if we are out pounding the pavement looking for a job, we're going to find employers who will not hire people with epilepsy. But we also discover that when we can let go of our own negative beliefs and perceptions, and not use them to limit us, doors open up to us. They do! One miraculously gets a waiter who is friendly and gives us excellent service. At the end of the meal, he shares with us that his brother is in a wheelchair, too. As a result he is comfortable with others challenged in this way. Similarly, we hear of an employer who has grown up in a family where there is epilepsy, and she is completely realistic about hiring people with this particular illness.

"I can't believe that!" said Alice.
"Can't you?" the queen said in a pitying tone. "Try
again, draw a long breath, and shut your eyes."
Alice laughed. "There's no use trying," she said. "One
can't believe impossible things."
"I dare say you haven't had much practice," said the
queen. "When I was your age, I always did it for half an
hour a day. Why, sometimes I've believed as much as six
impossible things before breakfast."

Lewis Carroll

While most people can recognize the value of identifying self-limiting beliefs and perceptions, it can be another matter to change them, to transform a negative to a positive. The transformation begins simply by knowing that what looks like the "truth"—that which appears to be "justified" by evidence in the real world—has its roots in the perceptions that we project into our lives. As we explore this insight, we begin to see that by changing our mind we can literally change our lives—or at least our experience of life.

Some of the ways people change their perceptions of the self-limiting aspects of an illness include searching for heroes and heroines with illness similar to their own who have been able to live successful and happy lives. You might find these people in books, movies, on television, or in real life. Keep your eyes and ears open for such heroes, and ask your family and friends to do the same.

We always learn from our perceptions by modeling other people and situations around us. We got our negative beliefs that way; it only stands to reason that we can change and adopt more positive ones the same way. An excellent place to begin changing our negative beliefs is with ourselves, of course, right here and now. You can begin with virtually any negative or self-limiting belief you might have about yourself. "Faith," said Buckminster Fuller, "is much better than belief. Belief is when someone else does the thinking."

Life Skill #9

While going through this material, take time to reflect on how your self-judgments or labels have affected decisions or choices you have made. For example, judging yourself unworthy because you are in a wheelchair, do you prevent yourself from going out to dinner? Are you afraid to ask old friends over for dinner because you must ask someone to cut up your food for you? In what ways are you limiting your activities by clinging to your negative self-judgments?

CHANGING NEGATIVE BELIEFS

I learned the way a monkey learns—by watching its parents.

Queen Elizabeth II

Begin by looking at a situation associated with your illness that is currently causing you stress, physical discomfort, or emotional distress. This situation could include physical symptoms and emotional, familial, financial, or behavioral concerns. For example, I found that I was becoming very frustrated, impatient, and discouraged about a weakness and shakiness I was experiencing in my legs when I went more than three hours without food. When this happened, I would become quite agitated. The more agitated I became, the more I blamed myself and my illness. Once the cycle started, my blaming mode picked up steam, linking up with all the negative beliefs and perceptions I associated with my illness; pretty soon, I was slipping into more general patterns of negative thinking, which originally had nothing to do with illness. Soon, what started as a simple discomfort had become the focal point for projections of all my darkest perceptions, dredged up from the archives as far back as my infancy.

Most of us have circumstances like this in our lives, whether we have an illness or not. Something does not fit our "pictures," frustrating or shaking us, and it becomes a magnet, drawing all our most uncomfortable perceptions to it. Pretty soon this magnet is attracting every negative belief and doubt that happens to be hovering around. In my case, with a tendency toward self-judgment and blame, I was soon immersed in a state of mind where I could see only the insecurities of my life.

FOSTERING THE QUALITIES OF MASTERSHIP

*It is common sense to take a method and try it. If it fails,
admit it frankly and try another. But above all,
try something.*

Franklin D. Roosevelt

I began to dissolve my habitual negative pattern by first acknowledging very simply and clearly what was happening at the moment. So, I wrote in my journal, "My legs feel weak and shaky whenever I miss meals or go without food for more than three hours."

Then I carefully recorded what I expected of myself during this time. Usually this came out in negative self-judgment and blame: "I should know better than to take a chance with my diet. What's wrong with me, anyway?"

Notice the disapproving tone here. It was with this feeling of unworthiness that I began projecting all my negativity about illness and my need to be perfect onto myself, my illness, Michael, and the world around me. It was like a dam bursting. However, with the next step in this exercise, I began turning this pattern around. Instead of limiting myself in this way, I asked a question—a very simple one, really: "What can I do or say to myself that is more self-supportive?" What could I tell myself the next time this situation arose? Here's the answer I recorded in my journal:

I will do my best to start each day with a large breakfast and vitamins. I will also keep nutritious snacks in my office so that I can maintain an even energy level throughout the day. I might even purchase a portable refrigerator for my office.

While changes like this may seem obvious once we've committed them to paper and put them into action, you'll be surprised at how many of the situations that really distress us about life start this way. So don't underestimate the power of this simple exercise! Here's how it looks step by step.

1. Note and describe symptoms or situations that trigger your self-judgment and blame.

2. Write down what you expect of yourself. Particularly pay attention to any ways you criticize yourself or get into negative judgments and self-talk.

3. Write down the ways you can think of to take positive action, as I did when I focused my attention on things I could do to maintain reasonable energy levels throughout the day.

If a situation comes to mind that doesn't seem to yield to this method, switch to a different one until you get one you can process this way. The main purpose of this exercise is not to immediately solve all your problems but to begin developing this new habit of cooperation with life *as it is*. Here you are taking full advantage of how perception and projection work in your life, particularly around issues associated with your illness, and are gaining experience in using that whole mechanism in a new way.

*Illness is telling us what we need to stop doing. If we look
at illness that way, then it has great value. It might be
telling us that we need to modify our work habits, to rest,
or to question what we are doing . . . It forces us to
reach out for help, bringing more love to us.*

O. Carl Simonton, MD

HOW YOU LEARNED TO BE SICK

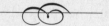

*I stopped believing in Santa Claus when my mother took
me to see him in a department store and he asked
for my autograph.*

Shirley Temple

As odd as it sounds, we have each received considerable training in
how to be sick. We have directly or indirectly been taught a complex set of emotional associations around what it means to be ill,
how we should relate to others when we are ill, and what we expect
of others. I developed the following beliefs as a result of my early
experiences with illness.

For example, in my childhood home I believed that getting ill
was an easy way of being cared for, getting attention, and feeling
close and loved.

I believe I received the message from my parents from an early
age that it was not safe to express emotions, so I learned to blink
back tears, brush off compliments, avoid eye contact, and shut out
the slightest ache or pain. I seldom expressed what I honestly felt,
and asking for what I really wanted was difficult indeed. Nobody
knew my pain.

I received an enormous amount of attention, however, whenever
I was sick. I felt loved, cared for, and safe when I was lying in bed
with a cold (real or imagined). Even today, I can remember looking
over at my bedside table, where everything to care for my cold had

been perfectly lined up. There was the cough syrup, the bottle of aspirin, the teaspoon, the washcloth, the glass of water, the thermometer, and the glass of juice. When I saw that, I just knew I was noticed and important. They were the artifacts that assured me everything was okay. I felt on top of the world—loved and appreciated, recognized for being me.

I especially liked it when my mother took my temperature, holding the thermometer up to the light to read it, shaking it down, placing it carefully under my tongue, sitting on the edge of my bed as she waited to read it again. I loved when she rubbed my chest with Vicks VapoRub to soothe a persistent cough. Her touch was gentle and caring as she wrapped my throat with a washcloth to insulate the penetrating heat. When I was sick was the only time that I remember being touched by her. Looking back on it—I must have been three or four—it seems obvious that these were tender moments where I perceived my mother feeling relaxed when she expressed her love for me. Here was a way she could safely show me that she cared and I could feel that I was important to her.

Those old perceptions hang on in the archives of my mind. I cannot say that this old way of being ill doesn't influence my life today. But the lessons I learned then have definitely gone through some important transitions. For example, if I had never looked at these childhood experiences I might have seen illness as the *only* way to experience being cared for and loved. And somewhere, very early on, I discovered that as an adult I wanted and could have much more than that—a relationship of openly giving, receiving, and growing, together. Where it still comes into play is in the unconditional care I provide myself. That is one of my mother's most valuable gifts to me. I make certain I have the supporting environment around me that will spiritually provide me with guidance and comfort. These standards and values planted the seeds for *You Are Not Your Illness*.

THE COURAGE TO HEAL

It is only with the heart that one can see rightly; what is essential is invisible to the eye.

Antoine de Saint-Exupéry

In the pages ahead, we'll be exploring memories of how we were treated as children when we were ill, as well as some of the more general memories that we might be projecting onto our illness today. Remember as you go along that these memories may provide important clues concerning your most important feelings, fears, and expectations about the role of illness in your life now. Like me, you might discover that you have an old perception that tells you that in order to be loved you have to be sick. And if you have lived with that vision for long, you will have probably bumped up against its limitations and are ready to seek more direct and positive ways of sharing your love. You can look at the old perception and say, "This is only one way of living my life; I can also fully express myself by giving and receiving the love I want in an infinite number of other ways."

My husband and my network of friends are open, generous, and emotionally expressive, providing experiences that are quite the opposite of what was available to me growing up. So, there is no need for me to use illness as a way of asking for love and attention. And believe me, my life is much richer, more exciting, and fuller because I learned not to limit myself to those early perceptions. I learned how to choose another way of looking at the world and participating in it.

It is important to note here that as we become increasingly aware of our limiting beliefs, and we learn to let go of them, they tend to fall away on their own. As we are in the process of changing, there are times when we may feel anxious or even empty. However, as we let one set of perceptions go, we make room for new ones that are much more attuned to the present. I cannot tell you how much more exciting my life became when I discovered how emotionally restricted I felt in my early life. So much opened up to me as I learned to trust the wisdom of my generous heart!

I can honestly say that illness has been my greatest teacher. It has not only taught me that I need not be ill to feel loved but has guided me in my growth psychologically as well as spiritually. I sometimes think it is like the ancient shamanic tradition wherein one learns to be a healer through being ill oneself. Somehow there's a wonderful irony in illness teaching us how to heal ourselves, be it in body, mind, or spirit.

CHILDHOOD WOUNDS AND ILLNESS

The needle that pierces may carry a thread that binds.

James Hastings

It is not easy to go back and remember painful events from the past. The problem is that old wounds, particularly those that are linked to our perceptions of illness, don't just evaporate into thin air. In most cases, we have to go back and take a moment to look closely at them before we can let them go.

There is a much-overused and much-misunderstood saying that goes, "We each create our own world." If we were to trace this idea back to its origin, we would probably discover that it is a distortion of Plato's famous cave analogy, in which we see early efforts to understand human perception. Assuming this is the case, we might more accurately say, "We each create how we *experience* the world."

Plato indicates that we can either look at the illusions of the shadows on the wall of the cave and become very frightened at the monsters we've created, or we can move toward the sunlight and find brightness and loving in the present moment.

When we start looking at the experience of illness, we perhaps do ourselves and others a great disservice by saying that we can perceive it any way we wish—that we can see everything about it as just wonderful and uplifting, if we would only make the effort. Clearly, disease isn't uplifting and wonderful. Who would not choose to live their lives without it? At the same time, it seems foolish to claim that our perceptions of illness are not strongly influenced by the perceptions we store in our minds. We really have far more choice about how we experience illness than we might think.

The mind is its own place, and in itself
Can make a Heaven of Hell, a Hell of Heaven.

John Milton

While there is no denying that physical pain and discomfort are nearly always associated with a serious, long-term illness, how we filter the experience of this pain through our perceptual minds, and interpret the perceptions we project will either make our lives unbearable or allow us to feel that our lives are worthwhile and valuable.

Given how our perceptions affect how we relate to illness, we can safely say that much of the pain we feel in the present is anchored in the past. Pulling up that anchor, by going back to where our emotions are still hanging on, allows us to break free from the past and move forward in the healing process. Just as an anchored boat can move around only within the range that its tether allows, so these old wounds allow us only limited progress in terms of our personal growth.

With illness as our focal point, take this opportunity to recall the different roles each of your caretakers played in your life. By caretakers, I mean anyone who was assigned the task of looking after you when you were small. Include anyone who had an impact on you as a child, whether it was a parent, a teacher, a minister, a doctor, a friend, a rabbi, or a distant relative. Use your journal to record your work in this area; you'll find it invaluable to have this information at your fingertips, allowing you to study any belief you are in the process of changing. Here are the key questions to ask yourself:

• What negative behaviors or painful events did you experience with your mother around illness?

Example: In my early life, the message I got, intended or not, was that I should be invisible. I came to believe that my emotions didn't count and were not important except at those times when I was ill.

- What negative behaviors or painful events did you experience with your father around illness?

  Getting sick definitely had getting attention as its reward. Until age eleven or so, I had asthma attacks every night. I didn't mind; I got the affection I wanted and needed. When I called for my dad to bring me juice or to help in some way, he always responded with kindness. When I called out to him, it became a game, knowing he was so attentive to my needs, as he lovingly cared for me.

- What negative behaviors or painful events around illness did you experience with others in your life—siblings, relatives, other caretakers?

  Remarks about my physical ability began to weaken my self-esteem and self-acceptance. I remember a relative calling me a klutz when I dropped things and making fun of my awkwardness in walking. I defended myself by saying, "But I slipped" or "it slipped," which then became a family taunt. I must have been only two or three years old.

As you recall these past experiences, please keep in mind that our first line of defense, particularly as children responding to the bewildering range of emotions we encounter, is to protect ourselves by shutting down our capacity to experience life. We numb ourselves. We choose not to feel, but are too young to realize that something is missing, something is wrong. This numbness does not go away just because we take ourselves out of the situation that caused us so much discomfort and pain. The way this pattern manifests itself later in our lives is that we say to ourselves, "Oh, that's all in the past. I don't have any feelings about that anymore." Indeed, because we have spent so many years numbing ourselves, our old wounds still cast a shadow, in the form of silence, anger, and hurt.

Rest assured that even if you have numbed yourself to these wounds, they continue to have a profound effect on you. Be kind to yourself. Stop rowing against the tug of the anchor. Pull the experiences to the surface once again so that you can feel what really happened to you and thus soothe and heal your pain.

The childhood shows the man,
As morning shows the day.

John Milton

Life Skill #10

With anger and with resentment (negative judgments against *other people* who don't live up to our expectations or who don't live up to our images about how *they* should be), we have *only one solution—change the image.* The images are ours. The anger is ours. When we realize that our anger is based not on our (or another's) *actions,* but on our *reactions* to our (or another's) actions, it's a day for celebration. Yet another thing we thought happened "out there" comes directly under our influence. We are learning to master and successfully live with our illness.

In childhood, we all do things just to survive. We naively adopt roles others want us to adopt, fearful that if we don't, we won't be loved and cared for. But as we take these survival techniques into our adult lives, we usually discover they cause pain we hadn't counted on. The best example I can offer is that in childhood I learned to be emotionally invisible in order to survive. Later in life, however, it became quite clear to me that in order to have the things I wanted in life, I'd have to become visible. Similarly, at the time I discovered I had MS, I had learned how to be visible and I was quite proud of myself for accomplishing this. I then became fearful that my illness would somehow make me numb again. I had to change these old beliefs and perceptions in order to even begin to live successfully with my illness.

Here are two examples of survival themes that ran through my life, with their benefits and consequences, followed by what I had to do to open up my locked-away, hidden, or forgotten feelings.

• In order to *survive* I had to shut out my feelings—so no one ever really listened to me. I was so successful at shutting out my feelings I barely knew they even existed.

- In order to *live* I needed to be creative and innovative—so I had to find my own voice and validate myself through my own journey of self-worth.
- In order to *survive*, I had to trust no one.
- In order to *live*, I had to learn how to trust others and myself enough to love and be touched emotionally by other people.

All of these applied to my perceptions of illness. And to live successfully with my illness, and not be invisible in the face of it, I had to apply the same healing principles I had applied to live in other areas of my life.

To better understand what's behind the survival patterns you have adopted, take a moment to identify negative feelings that you experienced over and over again in your relationships with each of your childhood caretakers: mother, father, others. These feelings can usually be described with single words, or perhaps lists of words —for example, resentful, embarrassed, insecure, sorrowful, joyless.

Other negative feelings you should note have to do with fear. These might include suspicious, worried, threatened, annoyed, anxious, nervous, terrified, paranoid, apprehensive, concerned.

In your journal, note all the feelings you associated with each caretaker, filling in with any stories or anecdotes that you feel might help you identify what went on in your childhood and why you feel as you do today.

Learning to be aware of feelings, how they arise and how to use them creatively, so they guide us to happiness, is an essential lifetime skill.

Joan Borysenko

On the following pages, I have provided lists of words describing different feelings, taken from the teachings of Harville Hendrix, Ph.D., in his breakthrough book *Getting the Love You Want: A Guide for Couples*. You might find these useful in doing the above work. As you reflect on your childhood relationships, simply go through the list and circle the words that strike a chord for you. Don't pause to mull over each word; rather, do it quickly, circling or underlining only those words that hold an immediate emotional or physical charge for you.

SAD

Sorrowful	Spiritless	Sullen
Downcast	Quiet	Moping
Dejected	Dark	Moody
Unhappy	Clouded	Glum
Willful	Vacant	Sulky
Depressed	Funereal	Empty
Melancholy	Mournful	Discontented
Gloomy	Dreadful	Discouraged
Cheerless	Dreary	Despondent
Somber	Flat	Hollow
Dismal	Dull	Disheartened
Joyless	Stricken	Sympathetic
Grieved	Downhearted	

ANGRY

Resentful	Irritated	Enraged
Furious	Annoyed	Inflamed
Incensed	Infuriated	Offended
Indignant	Irate	Envious
Worked up	Wrathful	Cross
Bitter	Virulent	Acrimonious
Boiling	Fuming	Defiant
Contentious	Belligerent	

HURT

Injured	Grieved	Offended
In pain	Distressed	Afflicted
Worried	Crushed	Mournful
Piteous	Woeful	Pathetic
Tortured	Agonized	In despair
Aching	Heartbroken	Victimized
Embarrassed	Tragic	

AFRAID

Fearful	Frightened	Timid
Chicken	Nervous	Anxious
Diffident	Fainthearted	Tremulous
Paralyzed	Shaky	Fidgety
Apprehensive	Immobilized	Restless
Aghast	Bewildered	Terrified
Panicky	Hysterical	Alarmed
Shocked	Horrified	Insecure
Worried	Doubtful	Suspicious
Hesitant	Irresolute	Dismayed
Awed	Cold	Scared
Trembling	Cowardly	Threatened
Menaced	Appalled	Petrified
Breathless		

DOUBTFUL

Cautious	Skeptical	Distrustful
Unbelieving	Suspicious	Uncertain
Dubious	Questioning	Wavering
Hesitant	Perplexed	Indecisive
Distant		

MISCELLANEOUS

Submissive	Dependent	Talkative
Seductive	Nauseated	Dominant
Abused	Powerless	
Tired	Too Busy	

In going through this list of words, noting those that seem to hold a charge for you, you may have noticed that the feelings you associate with your childhood are also prevalent when you think about your illness. It's important to recognize that all of these are reactions to events that occurred in your childhood. For the most part, they are learned perceptions, based on your earliest learned responses to your environment. For now, it is enough to know that they are perceptions and that therefore you can alter them.

Life Skill #11

When something happens that triggers a negative reaction in you, recognize it as an opportunity to pay attention to some part of yourself that you haven't accepted as yet. Shift the focus from the event to what is happening inside you. Check in with your body: feel where you are holding tension; notice your breathing; and notice the judgments you are making about what is happening.

LOVE IS LETTING GO OF FEAR

To suffer one's death and to be reborn is not easy.

Fritz Perls

One of the categories you dealt with in the above word-association section was fear. When we take the time to acknowledge our fears, and identify at least a little something about their source, we can begin to let them go. Because so much fear gets projected to our illnesses, it is particularly important to take a look at them. Here is a list of the most common fears, but feel free to add your own. (This list is adapted from the book *Living Beyond Fear* by psychologist Jeanne Segal, Ph.D.)

1. I fear the loss of love.
2. I fear losing any sense of my purpose and meaning in life.
3. I am afraid of progressive physical degeneration, loss of energy, or the further diminishment of other faculties.
4. I fear pain.
5. I fear the loss of status, my job, or career, I fear the loss of material possessions associated with this loss (for example, I am afraid I will not be able to pay the mortgage if I lose my job).
6. I fear that I will look foolish or ignorant.
7. I fear losing control of my life and becoming dependent on others.
8. I am afraid of dying.
9. I am afraid of the unknown or untried.
10. I am afraid of life's unpredictability.
11. I am afraid of success/failure.
12. I am afraid of being abandoned, both emotionally and physically.

If you want a place in the sun, you must leave the shade of the family tree.

Osage saying

Though we all experience some degree of fear of all the items on the list, as we look more closely at these fears, we discover that they begin to lose some of their charge. Certainly there are realities about having an illness that are not going to magically dissolve just because we look at these fears. But what we are seeking here is a shift of perception that allows us to be able to not be paralyzed or hypnotized by our fear. I think it takes courage to be a great warrior. The warrior is one who is not controlled by fear. The fear is there, surely, when the warrior's opponent comes rushing forward swinging a razor-sharp sword. But the well-disciplined warrior, rather than being motivated by fear, stays focused on what needs to be done to respond appropriately to the attack. Warriors place Light around them as a shield, making sure that what they do is an experience of truth and love. Remaining peaceful by placing love in their hearts, they have the mantle of the warrior around them. And the apprenticeship of the loving warrior is primarily getting to know fear in a way that the rest of us are not usually called upon to do—as one who serves with strength and purpose.

Since the goal of learning to live successfully with illness is primarily to be at peace with ourselves, the warrior analogy can be quite helpful to us here. In my personal process of self-exploration, it has been tremendously helpful to me to look at what frightens me most, as described above. When I look at the areas I want to avoid, I feel an inner peace, deep within my body and heart, believing, at last, as an adult, that I can handle them. This inner peace has become my foundation of safety as I move toward accepting my life just as it is right now. There is a stillness and peace that comes from within as I stay present in the moment, looking directly into the face of fear and loss.

RESPONSIBILITY AND LOVE—
FOUNDATIONS OF WELL-BEING

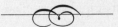

Experience is not what happens to a man. It is what a man does with what happens to him.

Aldous Huxley

Usually when we talk about responsibility, it is in terms of attempting to fix blame. I can still hear little voices from my childhood shouting, "Who's *responsible* for this?!" The real message here would be more accurately stated by asking, "Who's to blame for this?" But the kind of responsibility I'm talking about is a very different kind. My spiritual teacher, John-Roger, more accurately describes it as "being responsive." When using these words, he means "response-ability," the ability to respond in a constructive and appropriate way. This is the essence of the warrior mind. It is the kind of self-response-ability that says the following:

- I identify my real needs and find creative and supportive ways to meet them. For example, I now "walk" with my electric scooter so that I can participate in events that I find meaningful and uplifting. Or I ask friends to help me with meals when my husband is out of town on business.
- I stay in touch with my inner self, careful to pay attention to signals my body is giving me. For example, if I get a twinge in my stomach when I am about to eat a particular food, I stop and ask what this means. Usually I discover that my body knew I should not be eating that food that day.
- I explore every medical option I become aware of, sometimes asking for second and third opinions from specialists. I read books and articles, and attend or listen to taped lectures that deal specifically with my levels of interest.
- I inform myself of all current research. .
- I express myself directly, communicating to other people what I am experiencing in the moment.
- I realize the life I really want through loving, caring, sharing, touching, nutrition, exercise, and daily spiritual practices.

Take a moment now to think about and record in your journal ways that you can be a better "warrior" and remain responsive and open to the situations that in the past have caused you to be fearful.

FINDING SAFE HAVENS WITHIN US

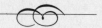

Reflect on your present blessings, of which every man has many, not on your past misfortunes, of which all men have some.

Charles Dickens

Even as you recall moments from your childhood that were frightening, you may also begin to recall safe havens that brought you comfort and allowed you to feel relatively free of your fears. Perhaps your safe haven was going to your room to read a book, or to hug a pet or favorite doll and "talk" to it about how you were feeling, or to listen to music. Many children also find safety and freedom from fear by engaging in physical activities, such as running, dancing, swinging on a swing, swimming, or skating. During such moments, they may actually enter an altered state where they feel quite calm and detached from the real world. You may have also had an actual place where you went to feel safe: a tree house in the backyard, the public library, a friend's house, or the room or home of a grandparent.

I always felt safe at the home of my next-door neighbor, "Aunt" Bea Pearlman, the mom of my childhood friend Joyce. I can still remember her brown-and-yellow flowered apple pattern dishes that she served my lunch on. I felt nurtured and taken care of, especially as she always knew how I liked grilled cheese sandwiches cooked for me, with the melted cheese dripping down the sides of the warm toast. She remembered how I liked it—compressed flat and cut in triangles that my seven-year-old "inner child," to this day, still refers to as "smiles."

For a moment, take the time to imagine yourself in that safe, warm place again, bringing back to your mind as many of the sensations associated with that place as you can. Whenever you recall something that makes you feel afraid, follow it up by recalling how you felt, what you saw, tasted, smelled, heard, and touched when you were in your safe place.

Don't underestimate the power of these nurturing positive memories. Just as you can recall and relive the negative ones, and stir up feelings of fear, you can also recall the positive ones, and experience feelings of safety and peace. When you have identified these safe havens, take a moment to record them in your journal. It has taken you a long time to develop the habit of shutting out negative feelings and it may take time to learn new, nurturing patterns of behavior. These memories are your antidotes to fear.

Life Skill #12

Start looking at the "ordinary" things in your life differently. Look at your home and your loved ones from a different perspective. Look at how you can alter everyday routines and begin to bring more variety into your activities. You might listen to a different radio station, or get out of bed from its opposite side, or experiment with different foods. Play with your perception of accepting and cooperating with alternative approaches that may reveal new opportunities of self-support for your present circumstances.

SELF-FORGIVENESS

Forgiveness is the only way to true health and happiness. By not judging, we release the past and let go of our fears of the future. In so doing, we come to see that everyone is our teacher and that every circumstance is an opportunity for growth in happiness, peace and love.

Gerald G. Jampolsky, M.D.

We hold so much against ourselves and against others; then we hold it against ourselves that we hold things against ourselves and others. The process of judging ourselves and others for not measuring up to our perceptions is a painful one. For this, forgiveness may be the greatest healer. Most people use the term *forgiveness* to accepting an apology or letting go of an old grievance for a past harm another person has done to you. We "forgive" a debt or we "forgive" a loved one who has said something hurtful. However, there is another meaning of forgiveness. It means letting go of your past perceptions. Forgiveness is unconditional. This includes forgiving ourselves.

To forgive is to be willing to let go of any hurt, guilt, or resentment that we feel in regard to another person—or ourselves. If we are holding on to a perception of self-blame, for example, emotionally beating ourselves up because of something we did or failed to do that we feel might have prevented the illness we have today, that perception accomplishes only one thing: it causes us stress. Similarly, if another person was in some way responsible for our present condition, we may be "holding a grudge." It is not unusual for one who has been seriously injured by another person's negligence to say, "I will never forgive her!" What we don't realize is that clinging to this past perception causes us pain and stress. To cling to it can never harm anyone but ourselves.

The fact that we did something or someone else did something is of little concern. The real problem for us began when we judged what happened as wrong, bad, mean, hurtful, nasty, improper, and so on. It's our judgment *against ourselves* we really need to forgive. The action was just the action. Our judgment that the action was bad, and so forth, is what caused our stress.

This is not the same as denying that the harmful situation happened or saying that it really doesn't matter. Certainly it matters! And you would do everything possible to avoid putting yourself in the position of getting injured again. But when we cling to blame or take the stance that we will "never forgive" the person who we feel is responsible for our pain, we are literally creating part of the "dis-ease" we wish to heal. Self-forgiveness is a promise to yourself that you will not cause yourself any further pain by clinging to these perceptions, as if by doing so you were punishing the other person (or yourself.) Our lack of forgiveness in such situations is, in fact, part of the disease—and we can heal it. We do this by recognizing that blame (and self-blame) is a specific kind of perception that we can let go of, thus freeing ourselves from its painful grasp.

SELF-FORGIVENESS IS AN INNER PROCESS

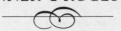

Without forgiveness life is governed by an endless cycle of resentment and retaliation.

Roberto Assaglioli

Forgiveness is always self-forgiveness. It does not require the participation of anyone else. The process is a simple one.

To forgive yourself, begin by saying the following:

- "I forgive myself for holding on to those perceptions that cause me pain." (To me, this means I will release myself from negative perceptions.)

- "I forgive my parents [or others] for being emotionally repressive." (To me, this means "I will let go of any blame I feel toward my parent. Who I am today is my responsibility.")

YOU ARE NOT YOUR ILLNESS / 112

Sometimes, when people learn that they have a serious illness, they begin judging themselves for not seeking medical help sooner, before the disease had progressed to the present stage. Again, it is *your judgment* that the action was wrong, the action itself is not the issue, at this point.

- Tell yourself, "I forgive myself for not seeing a doctor sooner." (To me, this means, "I will forgive myself for anything I did or did not do in the past. Instead, I will be responsive to life in the present as I remember who I am.")

Any of the fears or other negative self-judgments you may have uncovered in this chapter are opportunities for your forgiveness. Forgive yourself for judging, knowing it was the judgment—not the action—that caused the pain, hurt, and separation. Remember, you are not saying that it does not matter that you or another person did something to cause your present pain. But that was then, and this is now. Unhook yourself from the past so that you can be at peace with your life today.

She got even in a way that was almost cruel. She forgave them.

Ralph McGill (about Eleanor Roosevelt)

Life Skill #13

The forgiveness phrases on page 111 and above are always available to you whenever you need them. Practice them often. All upset is caused by our judgment of a situation. Forgive the judgment, and the upset tends to fade.

UNTIE YOURSELF

If thou art pained by an external thing, it is not this thing that disturbs thee, but thy own judgment about it. And it is in thy power to wipe out this judgment now.

Marcus Aurelius

Many people have found it helpful to imagine their fears, judgments, and negative beliefs tied to them by a long length of rope. You might see these negative perceptions contained in a huge box or a heavy burlap sack, or some other container. As you go through the day, you are forced to drag these containers along with you, constantly tugging at the rope to pull them along. What a burden it is, until you make the decision to release yourself.

To forgive or let go, just imagine that you stop pulling the fears, beliefs, and grievances behind you. You turn around, grab hold of the rope, reach inside your pocket, and produce a sharp knife. Then with one slice you cut through the rope. Ah, at last you are free! You need no longer carry that burden. Now say good-bye to your past perceptions!

If you like to work with visual images, draw a picture of this process of cutting the rope that binds you to your past perceptions, or come up with your own image of physically releasing yourself from a burden.

POSITIVE FOCUSING VERSUS POSITIVE THINKING

The greater part of our happiness or misery depends on our dispositions and not on our circumstances.

Martha Washington

As you draw to the end of this chapter, begin to turn your attention from the negative events of your past and focus on the positive. Practicing this focus will help you be more receptive to the present.

But be advised about "positive thinking" that actually disguises a kind of emotional tyranny. Let me take a moment to explain.

If you are anything like me, you probably have well-meaning friends who urge you to think more positively about your illness or physical condition. "Let go! You don't need your illness," they might say. Others might say, "What do you gain by holding on to your illness?" People want you to heal faster because of their own discomfort with what's happening to you.

Be careful of those who put pressure on you this way. They may be doing it out of sincerity and love, but I urge you to ignore their efforts. Their insistent concerns may reinforce your own patterns of guilt, shame, or embarrassment over the fact that you haven't instantly healed yourself. Recognize that what they are expressing is their own helplessness; they would like you to be completely well right now.

Assure yourself that you are doing the very best you can. Be gentle with yourself and respect your own pace. The old clichés of thinking positively, or holding positive visualizations in your mind, do not encompass the fact that there are strong underlying feelings that you need to heal. You do not instantly and miraculously heal a wound that you have been carrying since childhood—at least not by simply creating a positive image. As we've seen in this chapter, we sometimes need to literally go back and relive the experience before we can unhook ourselves from it.

NEW AGE GUILT

When some people first discover how powerful thoughts are, they begin worshipping the mind the way some people worship God. They deny the truth of what's actually happening for a mental image they find more pleasant. This creates a separation between the positive thinker and his or her reality.

John-Roger

Something I call New Age guilt is rampant in our society today. This starts with a distortion of the concept that we each create our own worlds, which we discussed previously. New Age guilt goes a step further, saying, "We each create our own illnesses." If you look closely enough, you begin to see that there is a peculiar kind of arrogance in such statements, as if this person's ego is so enormous that it believes it and only it is somehow in charge of the world. The ego, of course, is very good at that, convincing us that we are safe only if we allow it to run things.

We know that most illness has varied and complex "causes." A few of these may be factors that we can consciously control—such as not smoking, because tobacco has been shown to significantly add to the chances of getting certain kinds of cancer. But there are other factors, over which we have little or no control—genetics, environmental pollution, accidents, events that occurred when you were still in your mother's womb, and so on.

New Age guilt begins with the premise that you can figure out what you are gaining from your illness, what your disease means to you. Then, you are supposedly "empowered" to let it go and no longer be its victim. But, once again, this search for "meaning" and motive is a little like the scientist who presumes that he can dis-cover the meaning of the universe. As Susan Sontag says in her book *Illness as Metaphor*, "Nothing is more punitive than to give a disease meaning—that meaning being invariably a moralistic one."

This is not to say that we can't be *positively focused*. We all know the lesson of having a choice between seeing our cup as half full or seeing it as half empty. Similarly, we can look out the window on a rainy day and say, "Oh, too bad it's raining. It's so dark and horrible outside." Or we can light a fire in the fireplace, put on our favorite music, and use the day to catch up on our paperwork or to read a good book. These are examples of positive focusing.

Positive thinkers (as distinguished from positive focusers) tend to be characterized as boundlessly optimistic, setting and holding on to unrealistic goals, totally ignoring their current life situation. I've heard women who are still in physical therapy saying, "I am going to run a marathon next year," when walking to the ladies' room is still a challenge. At best, this is wishful, hopeful thinking. At worst, it is a sophisticated form of denial that literally separates people from themselves and from dealing appropriately with where their lives are today.

What happens to those of us who aren't healed after hours upon hours of visualization, meditation, and positive thinking? I got one answer to that question from a friend of mine with MS, who said, "If I had only thought more positively about my illness, I would have gotten better by now!" She ended up blaming herself for having this disease, still holding on to the perception that she had total control of it.

It takes courage to remember that our love for ourselves, *not our judgments of ourselves*, is the most important part of our healing journey. There are no "shoulds" in illness. Improvement or decline has many influences. Be aware that you are not to blame if the course of your illness does not unfold according to your own plan. Be gentle with yourself. Always be gentle.

LOVING YOURSELF WELL

The sun will set without Thy asistance.

The Talmud

With the above points in mind, let's close this chapter by practicing positive focusing, as distinct from positive thinking. Do this by focusing your attention on your own best qualities. In your journal, think about words and concepts such as "creative, honest, enthusiastic, reliable, romantic, courageous, considerate, understanding, kind, grateful, appreciative, vulnerable, dedicated, tender, determined, or funny," rather than your "beautiful red hair, blue eyes, or wonderful figure."

Whenever negative thoughts or self-judgments come up, challenge them with this more positive focus on yourself. From time to time, take a look at the beliefs and perceptions you are holding in your mind about yourself. Note if you are holding on to guilt or blame; look at ways to heal these feelings through letting go of any negative attachments you have toward people or situations in the past.

Look at the source of your beliefs, feelings, and perceptions, with the realization that you can change and transform them. And keep your focus on learning to love yourself well. That is ultimately the central goal of all healing.

Sweet are the uses of adversity, which like the toad,
ugly and venomous, wears yet a precious jewel in his
head.

William Shakespeare

Remember that all the perceptions that we project onto ourselves
or to the world also go into forming how we experience our illnesses.
As you change your perceptions, and as you learn to balance any
inner disturbance by letting go (forgiving) of those perceptions that
cause you pain and discomfort, you will begin to notice that how
you relate to your illness changes. It is so easy to think of the illness
itself as being the "cause" of all the dark associations we have
around it, or to blame it for our not being able to be "whole" or to
live our lives fully. But when we shift our perceptions, we realize we
are free to be whole and live successfully with our illness.

Positive attitudes—optimism, high self-esteem, an
outgoing nature, joyousness, and the ability to cope with
stress—may be the most important bases for continued
good health.

Helen Hayes

In the next section of the book, Part Two, The Challenge, we begin
to look at how we change and who we become when we change our
relationship with ourselves, the world around us, and our illness.

The purpose is not to identify with the body which is
falling away, but with the consciousness of which
it is a vehicle.

Joseph Campbell

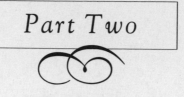

Part Two

THE
CHALLENGE

Life doesn't meet you halfway;
you have to meet life all the way.

Gurudev (Yogi Amrit Desai)

4

How We Change

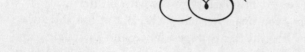

SHIFTING OUR PERCEPTIONS INTO EACH NEW MOMENT

And a woman spoke, saying, "Tell us of Pain." And he said. "Your pain is the breaking of the shell that encloses your understanding."

Kahlil Gibran

There is probably not a single person with a serious, debilitating illness who would not choose to be able-bodied and well if given the choice. Who would not trade illness for health, or a palsied hand for a steady one? Surely, for as long as I am here in a physical body, I will seek comfort and health. But as we begin to grasp the role of perception and open ourselves to experience our feelings, there are other questions we must begin to ask. I begin to ask what is my life about right now, in this exact moment in time? And *what can I change* that will make it full and rich, notwithstanding my prognosis or the fear, regret, blame, or other discomfort that I meet again with each new day? What is my life about now that I cannot even stand, now that I cannot even make dinner for my husband or go to the bathroom alone?

Whenever I find myself pondering such questions, I invariably remember *Beauty and the Beast,* one of my favorite childhood fairy tales. For me, the story has taken on a special meaning. It has become a heartfelt metaphor for my illness. For me, Beauty is goodness, health, compassion, love, and freedom, while the Beast is fear, pain, grief, enslavement, and illness.

In the traditional story, Beauty, the young princess, chooses to leave behind the comfort and protectiveness of her castle home to live with the Beast. At first Beauty resists with all her heart. It is difficult for her to even imagine such a fate. But at last she knows that she must go beyond her own resistance and incredulity and look squarely at the problem she is facing. The cost of failing to do this is nothing short of her father's death. Noble, loving, and loyal, she cannot allow her father to sacrifice his life for her happiness, so she leaves her home to live with the Beast.

The Beast turns out to be even more hideous-looking than she had feared. Night after night, she can barely work up the courage to be in his presence. Only by drawing from her own inner resources —her dedication to goodness, courage, and love—is she able to stay with the monster.

Time passes, and little by little, Beauty's heart is moved by the Beast. She sees his suffering, feels his longing for love, made so impossible by a physical appearance that repulses others and causes them to flee from him. She comes to genuinely care for him. She comes to know and appreciate his vulnerability and tenderness, which lie well hidden behind his rough exterior.

The Beast falls ill, and as he lies dying, Beauty comes to him. As she sits at his side, administering to what could be his last needs, she is moved by a deep love she feels for him. Magically, as if revived by her love, the Beast stirs. At last, no longer separated by the fears and repulsion that have kept them separated during all their time together, they are moved by what they feel in their hearts.

Beauty and the Beast embrace, and in the next sweet and touching moments, they kiss. Instantly, the Beast is transformed. Through the alchemy of his and Beauty's love he becomes a handsome prince. Love has unlocked his true beauty, the physical form now mirroring his true spirit, which previously was impossible for others to see. And, as in all romantic fairy tales, the two marry and live happily ever after.

This uplifting fable becomes a powerful metaphor for anyone living with a serious illness. It is a reminder to us that change comes when we acknowledge the painful and frightening emotions (the Beast) with which we live daily. And it is a reminder that through love (Beauty) we can transform (change) all that we consider dark and forbidding. Healing our lives begins with acknowledging both the Beauty and the Beast within ourselves.

Be willing to have it so acceptance of what has happened is the first step to overcoming the consequences of any misfortune.

William James

In his book *The Uses of Enchantment: The Meaning and Importance of Fairy Tales*, Bruno Bettelheim makes the point that it is impossible to destroy the dark side of our personalities—the Beast that lives in all of us. There are parts we would like to deny, of course, parts we push away and do not want to admit are there. Bettelheim states that the main prerequisite to change is learning to accept and embrace what in the past we have found unacceptable about ourselves. Out of this acceptance comes profound compassion for ourselves and others. Out of it come new levels of personal integrity, and human strengths that fuel our forward movement toward a deeper understanding and appreciation for our lives. As the shadow comes forth into the light, we discover a new source of personal power that helps us through even the most trying days. We discover that what we thought was our greatest adversary, and something that we must resist and avoid, now becomes our greatest ally.

Watch a man in times of . . . adversity to discover what
kind of man he is; for then at last words of truth
are drawn from the depths of his heart, and
the mask is torn off.

Lucretius

More and more, even as my legs lose strength and my hand grows less firm, I am able to meet and embrace my deepest fears—to, in effect, live peacefully with my Beast. And as this occurs, I recognize significant changes occurring in the way I relate to my illness and my life. I find new depths of courage to face shadows that in the past filled me with terror or disgust, or that brought out my most defensive denials. And I find unexpected ways of viewing even new physical difficulties I may be having. I must confess there are still many times when I feel abandoned by Beauty and when I lose all patience and understanding for the Beast. When this happens all my fear and hurt, my unsupportive thoughts and habits of denial, become the real Beast, oppressing and enslaving me. Envy, bitterness, anger, and jealousy drown out my joy, casting shadows across my heart. I become a prisoner of my own making.

Trust in God, but tie your camel to a tree.

Arab proverb

This process of change is a time to acknowledge, experience, and then put aside our deepest fears, our feelings of sadness, prejudice, pain, anger, and grief. We are, quite literally, healing ourselves by liberating ourselves from those enslavements that "warp the Spirit and blight the mind, that destroy the Soul even though they leave the flesh alive. For men can be enslaved in more ways than one."

Those words are taken from a translation of the *Haggadah*, the Jewish book of prayer that is a centerpiece of the Passover celebration. Passover illustrates how we bring about or allow change in our lives. During Passover, we are called upon to be free from the tyranny of self-centeredness. Passover is a rededication to the struggle for freedom and to our healing on all levels that acknowledge the importance of the kind of transformational process we see depicted in the fable *Beauty and the Beast*. This story illustrates all the steps necessary for negotiating even the most difficult changes in our lives.

FROM DESPAIR TO INTEGRITY

If we had no winter, the spring would not be so pleasant;
If we had not sometimes taste of adversity,
prosperity would not be so welcome.

Anne Bradstreet

When we have an illness, we are constantly forced to *embrace the Beast*, sometimes when it is at its most fearsome and we are not ready to look beyond the surface of the horrors we must face. It is at times such as these that we are most in need of those skills required for lasting change.

In 1990, I planned a spiritual pilgrimage to Egypt and Israel. I had a vision of myself sailing down the Nile. Mine would be a journey of faith, courage, endurance, and the power of tenacity to ultimately conquer all. With my sturdy walking cane, my wheelchair, and my undauntable panache, nothing could stop my determined passage into antiquity—not the 110-degree heat, the dusty conditions, the unfamiliar food, the scarcity of bathrooms, or the steep and demanding trek to many of the places I was determined to visit.

Anticipating my journey for over a year, I drove myself hard. In my blind fervor to get well, I stopped listening inwardly. Then, quite abruptly, it seemed that all my efforts to heal my body began doing just the opposite. A special diet I was on to eliminate food allergies and chemical sensitivities sharply reduced my tolerance for any food whatsoever. I dropped down to a mere one hundred pounds. At a well-known hospital rehabilitation program, I had an allergic reaction to an experimental injection of phenol; meant to improve my gait, it made matters much worse. During this alternative treatment I developed a severe bladder infection, necessitating further hospitalization; in the treatment that followed, I had a life-threatening reaction to the medication. But it did not stop there. Increased spasms in both my feet made it increasingly difficult for me to walk, even with my cane and braces. I developed a new tremor in my left hand. And finally, with an administrative decision to end gait training and swimming sessions, my legs quickly became too weak to endure any further therapy appointments of the pre-scribed rehabilitation program.

There could be no doubt that these physical problems had to be dealt with. But beyond that, there were other issues at which I really had to take a long and careful look. As one who had always lived with the perception that *productivity*—doing and being active—was the only real measure of one's worth, I had also believed that I was nothing if I couldn't be in control of my own destiny. I had little tolerance for my life going any way other than what I intended. I believed in having it all—but had never stopped to ask myself what I really meant by that.

All my planning to go to Egypt and Israel, all my dreams of sailing victoriously down the Nile, suddenly came to an abrupt, heart-shattering end. I could no longer fool myself; my body simply was not strong enough to endure such a journey. Humbled by the reality of the challenging trip and my extreme physical weakness, Michael and I canceled our plans. And upon doing so I collapsed into despair.

THREE STEPS FORWARD, THREE STEPS BACKWARD

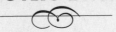

*Learn to wish
that everything should come to pass
exactly as it does.*

Epictetus

Surely, this was change—but not what I'd been consciously seeking. However, it did not take long for me to recognize the beginnings of a new transformation, like a tiny seed pushing out its first tendrils through the soil. The change that emerged surprised and challenged me in ways I would never have anticipated. What's more, it became clear to me that my perception about productivity being the measure of a person's worth—which was so central to my thinking—was not going to help me out of my current despair. In fact, it was slowly dawning on me that perhaps this point of view was more the cause than the cure! When I saw this, I at first felt more despairing than ever. If I could no longer measure my own life and others' this way, what was I left with? Where would I find a sense of meaning and purpose? Then I remembered something the psychologist Erik Erikson had once said about dignity and integrity: "The possessor of integrity is ready to defend the dignity of his own lifestyle against all physical and economic threats." At first, I wasn't sure why this was significant for me, but as I questioned it I started getting clearer.

I had always seen myself as a person of integrity, and in the face of the challenges I now confronted I drew encouragement from Erikson's words. I could choose despair or I could choose dignity and integrity. But what exactly did this mean to me? How did it reflect on the changes I was facing at this time? I began to take a hard look at all the parts of my life, particularly at what I most resisted examining—my fear, my insecurity, my pain, my grief. I began listening more carefully to my inner child and to the spiritual guidance whose voice seemed to be growing in strength. I don't think I had ever been more honest with myself. This, I realized, was the integrity Erikson was talking about, the integrity with which I would regain my dignity. This was to be the real key to successfully negotiating the emerging changes.

LIVING IN PRESENT TIME

The secret of a warrior is that he believes without believing. . . . To just believe would exonerate him from examining his situation. A warrior, whenever he has to involve himself with believing, does it as a choice.

Carlos Castañeda

Inspired by Erikson, I forced myself to look at all that I'd been denying about my life. I realized, for the first time, that everything I found difficult to acknowledge in myself had a common denominator: fear. My grief, hopelessness, terror and rage, my need to control others, and my overwrought anxiety did not spring spontaneously from my physical condition but were the products of my resistance to facing my fears. It isn't easy separating illness from the thoughts, feelings, and behavior we bring to it, of course. Certainly illness and losing one's physical capacities seem to *justify* reactions such as grief, rage, and hopelessness. But just as with any challenges we might have to face, it is these greatest personal trials that call upon us to look deeply into ourselves, to come to terms with the perceptions that shape how we experience the world and be open to whatever change might bring us peace of mind.

Following a path of integrity, I began to see how I had used denial in relation to my illness—employing various deceptions to make me look good, such as covering my left hand to prevent others from noticing its uncontrollable tremors. I also began to see how my need to control, driven by my fear, came out in efforts to manipulate others, to always have the last word, and in behaviors that smacked of emotional abuse. I was reminded of what so many great teachers have said, that when we begin to look at aspects of ourselves that we would rather disown, we begin to see how the denial actually increases the fear and pain we are trying to escape. To change means looking squarely at the thing we most vehemently deny.

INTEGRITY: FORMULA FOR SUCCESS

Integrity is having the courage to go with the truth as you know it, as a heartfelt response with care and consideration for others.

John-Roger

For periods of time, as I followed this path of integrity and dedicated myself to giving up the old behaviors, I found myself feeling defenseless and fearful. At times those feelings have been extremely uncomfortable. But out of these periods of defenselessness I am now beginning to discover a new source of strength, one that is far more fruitful and fulfilling than my previous perceptions. I am reminded of the phrase "perfect vulnerability is perfect protection." As I learn the power of this defenselessness, I find in myself a willingness to share my vulnerability as well as my strength; out of this there continues to evolve a heartfelt courage to move forward. Experiencing and embracing what I once denied about myself have allowed me to tap into the deep spiritual essence we all share and which can carry us beyond our sadness and grief, beyond our deepest fears and frustrations.

AWAKENING INTO LIGHT: SECRETS OF SUCCESSFUL CHANGE

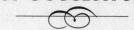

Many lessons continue to evolve from the experiences I've had following the cancellation of our trip to Egypt. One of the most important for me has been around a new understanding of change itself. Life is constant change. In resisting change, we literally resist life. Instead of fearing change and guarding ourselves from it, we begin to heal and reclaim our lives when we embrace it. If there is a single goal in learning how to successfully handle change, it is that. When I am at my best, I actively seek challenges rather than run from them. Since I apparently do not have the option of instantly eliminating my physical and emotional pain, I have accepted them as my teachers. They spur me on to honest self-exploration, expanding the opportunities for loving acceptance of myself. They guide me beyond my resistance, showing me a more direct path toward increased energy, enthusiasm for living, compassion for others, and love.

SEVEN PRINCIPLES TO FREEDOM AND INNER PEACE

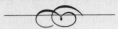

As to me I know of nothing else but miracles.

Walt Whitman

In the remaining pages of this chapter, you will find the Seven Keys for Personal Change that I developed and practiced in my own experiences with meeting the challenges of illness and living successfully with them. In using these seven principles, you can move forward on the journey that defines your healing path. There are few days I do not turn to them for help in charting the unpredictable course that my illness is constantly presenting to me.

Briefly, the seven personal keys are: (1) Honesty; (2) Acceptance; (3) Patience; (4) Observation; (5) Compassion; (6) Cooperation; (7) Loyalty. To better understand what these are and how they can help us live successfully with illness, let's take a look at how they were employed in the *Beauty and Beast* fable and in my own story of my canceled trip to Egypt.

1. HONESTY

When we are no longer able to change a situation, we are challenged to change ourselves.

Viktor Frankl

What is honesty? My definition of honesty means letting go of illusions, pretensions, and judgments and having the courage to face my life exactly as it is right now. It is how we are with ourselves when we are living most successfully and fully in the moment.

In the *Beauty and the Beast* story, Beauty at first resists even the thought that she would have to go and live with the Beast, whom she finds terrifying and repulsive. She is incredulous, every cell of her being rejecting such a fate. In this state of resistance and denial, she cannot look at this reality long enough to make even the first step toward a solution. At last, pushed by the realization that her father's life depends on her decision, she looks squarely and un-flinchingly at *what is*, letting go of her dreams of how things *ought to be*. At this point she is taking her first step toward successful change.

In my own story of canceling my trip to the Middle East, I made my first step toward genuine change when I looked unflinchingly at my weakened physical condition and then at the grueling challenge of the journey. It was when I began to see the dire consequences of measuring my self-worth only by my productivity, which at that time meant frantically rushing around from one specialist to an-other, for a different brace, a sturdier cane, the safety of a folding walker, or the next claim of a miracle cure. Honesty helped me see *the way it is* and move toward the inner freedom that comes with genuine acceptance. It allowed me to see that I would not be the same person, physically—and it allowed me to accept that fact. Through honesty, we stop trying to control the present; we stop trying to stop change. Through honesty we rededicate ourselves to building a quality of life for ourselves from what we have right here and now. Honesty takes great courage, to be sure. But role models and heroes in this arena abound.

I know God will not give me anything I can't handle,
I just wish that He didn't trust me so much.

Mother Teresa

Matisse, Christy Brown, and Renoir could not have accomplished what they did without taking that first step toward change—hon-esty. Only by doing so were they able to find ways to realize quality lives that fully honored the power and depth of the human spirit. Honesty was my first step in unmasking myself, stripping away the veils and getting to know my dark side. In doing so, I found new freedom from that part of me that measured the worth of myself and others by their productivity. Out of this came new clarity—that to find compassion and love for oneself and others could be profoundly healing, celebrating the human spirit. Honesty serves the purpose of moving us through this physical world with greater ease and harmony.

2. ACCEPTANCE

And that's the way it is.

Walter Cronkite

Acceptance is the ability to let go of our perceptions of how things *should be* and let in the reality of *what is*. It is the ability to open ourselves up to *what is*, which makes it possible for us to take action based on that reality rather than one that exists only in our minds.

When Beauty goes to live with the Beast, her repulsion and horror at first keep her at a distance. Based on perceptions of beauty that she holds in her mind, Beauty cannot look beyond the Beast's physical appearance and rough manners. Slowly, however, she lets go of her preoccupations with what constitutes an aesthetically pleasing companion and an acceptable lifestyle; this is the turning point, when *acceptance* replaces judgment and she starts to let the Beast into her life exactly as he is, not just as she'd like him to be. Interestingly, this is when her life with him begins to improve.

In my own case, it was at the point just beyond my despair that I took steps toward acceptance. As difficult as it was to accept the fact that my body was too weakened to survive the trip to the Middle East, it brought me into a higher quality of life than I perhaps had ever known. I discovered that my acceptance brought forth a brand new level of self-support, compassion, and love. In a very real way, I replaced my productivity-oriented, "I'll show them all" attitude, which sailing down the Nile symbolized for me, with what for me was a new, uplifting inner journey where I discovered the comfort of compassion and love for myself and others.

Acceptance takes practice. I coach myself in this practice by reminding myself that I only need to *surrender to the present moment, accepting one moment at a time*. I only need to accept my own thoughts, even those that I feel are negative or judgmental. I accept everything around me, remembering that I don't have to like it or agree with it. I only need to accept that these things are present, existing in the here and now. Accepting the tremor in my hand or my low tolerance for the medicine I am given to control it has been anything but easy. But this practice in acceptance has helped me become more comfortable with my illness. I do not mean to imply that we can become accepting by waving some kind of magic wand. On the contrary, I have often said that the challenge of acceptance is simple—but far from easy.

Avoid holding on to rigid points of view—as in "I've got it; this is it; I accept no other way that works." Rather, you might say, "This way is working right now." And if it's working ten minutes from now, *accept it* and keep working with it. But if it stops working, move on to something else, because it will no longer be honest and true for you.

There is no good in arguing with the inevitable. The only argument available with an east wind is to put on your overcoat.

James Russell Lowell

---

3. PATIENCE

Patience is enjoying the journey. It's not climbing the mountain to get to the top; it's climbing the mountain to enjoy the climb. Enjoy the process of your own life.

John-Roger

Most of us spend a considerable portion of our lives believing we must respond immediately to our first impressions and judgments in any situation. We rarely pause long enough to wonder how much the problem we are experiencing is the result of our own perceptions. Nor do we give ourselves an opening to ask if our experience might be vastly improved by perhaps finding another way of looking at that situation.

Certainly, Renoir had to go through a perceptual shift in order to find a new way to paint. Had he held on to a rigid point of view and said, "No, there is only one way to paint, only one style, only one way to hold the brushes, and I will not accept any other," he never could have painted some of his greatest works. As he looked honestly at his situation, coming into a place of accepting the truth, and then *being patient* with himself and his situation, his solution emerged.

We find the magic of patience expressed also in the *Beauty and the Beast* story, with Beauty taking a watch-and-see approach (the very essence of patience) that allowed her to discover the love she and the Beast would eventually share.

In my own situation, canceling my trip to Egypt and then being patient with my own process led me to make new discoveries about myself, ones that opened up a new and joyous way of relating to the world. I was able to stop measuring myself and others according to my perception that our self-worth is dependent wholly on productivity. As you enter the areas of honesty, acceptance, and patience and learn to flow with *that which is,* you may start to feel a stillness within you, a stillness that will allow you to tap into the fourth personal key—observation.

The clouds pass and the rain does its work, and all individual beings flow into their forms.

I Ching

---

4. OBSERVATION

You do not need to leave your room. Remain sitting at your table and listen. Do not even listen, simply wait. Do not even wait, be quiet, still and solitary. The world will freely offer itself to you to be unmasked, it has no choice, it will roll in ecstasy at your feet.

Franz Kafka

Much of the time, we go around looking at the world as if through a series of personal filters. We see only what we're looking for, and we take in only what we wish to take in. We have certain perceptions about what is beautiful, what is difficult, what is dangerous, what kinds of situations we find pleasing and acceptable, and what sorts of things we find objectionable. When we observe certain signals or signs, we immediately reject the situation and refuse to go any further with it—or we at least become guarded and resistant.

Observation requires us to suspend our personal filters, if only for an instant, and simply take in what is there. Beauty, in going to live with the Beast, at first sees only ugliness, and is repulsed and frightened by it. However, as she learns, a little at a time, to suspend her judgments and just *observe* what's there, she begins to see the Beast's pain and vulnerability. She opens up to his humanness, and as she does this she experiences her own life as deeply fulfilling.

Many experts in human behavior, all through the ages, have said that we do not really learn how to love either ourselves or others until we learn the art of observation. We do not even become aware of the "others" in our life until we stop limiting our experience by looking at them only through our own perceptual filters.

Meditation is one of the best ways we have available for learning to observe. It allows you to see all sorts of new possibilities, concepts, and ideas. During meditation, we slow down or stop the mental activity that ordinarily goes into perception and judgment of ourselves and the world around us. For the period we are meditating, we become very quiet within. The memory of the inner peacefulness we experience in this way can be carried over into the challenge of illness, allowing us to open up to new ways of seeing our lives.

Be here now.

Ram Dass

I look at my shaking left hand and watch it as an observer. I remember the life of Christy Brown with admiration and respect. Could I build my life from this moment, *right now*, as if this were the only truth I ever knew? Does it matter how I walk, or if my vision gets blurry, or my speech slurred? Why should I not accept and love myself and others as we are right now—warts, tremors, and all? Could I live without the goal of getting well? Could I still research my options and take care of myself without that obsession, without that attachment? Could I abandon my despair and yield completely to acceptance? These self-supportive questions and insights allow me, for a while, to love myself authentically and with no judgment.

Be witness to it, rather than a reactor to it.

Gurudev (Yogi Amrit Desai)

---

5. COMPASSION

To believe in God is impossible—
not to believe in Him is absurd.

Voltaire

For most of us, compassion is something we feel for other people—and when faced with serious illness, we may at first be so focused on ourselves that we lose sight of everything else. We want others to feel compassion and understanding for us, to be sure, but it may not be immediately apparent how our own compassion can assist in our healing.

What's important to remember is that the healing power of compassion begins with forgiving ourselves. Until I could say, "I forgive myself for judging myself as unworthy of God's love," I could neither feel others' compassion for me nor extend it to others.

Compassion is the ability to see how it all is.

Ram Dass

We see in *Beauty and the Beast* how Beauty allowed herself to be vulnerable to the Beast's pain, which allowed her to discover first compassion and then love. But with an illness, our compassion usually begins with recognizing inner parts of ourselves, which can be quite elusive. I discovered my own compassion when I shifted my focus of attention from seeking out authorities who might somehow help me control or cure my illness to paying more attention to my inner child. Like an orphan cast into the hostile streets, my inner child cried out for my attention, frightened and terribly disillusioned with how life had turned out for her. In the beginning, I hadn't wanted to listen to her, didn't want to hear her. "Why bother hearing her sob her grief and scream her terror?" I reasoned. I was too busy to listen, too intent on looking for answers in the outer world.

As I began, more and more, to listen to myself, and to experience compassion for myself, much of my frantic search for answers outside myself ceased. As I experienced deeper compassion for myself, facing my fears and disappointments, I discovered that I could drop many of my defenses and self-judgments. I began to see beyond the roles and "rackets" I played in an effort to feel safe. I began to cradle the disowned parts of myself in the safety of my own self-care, reclaiming parts of myself I had abandoned many years before. Meeting the challenge of illness enables us to just keep simplifying, forgiving, and moving forward into each new moment.

Your vision will become clear only when you can look into your own heart. Who looks outside, dreams; who looks inside, awakes.

Carl Jung

The compassion I experience today is healing for me in so many ways it is almost impossible to name them all. Through our compassion for ourselves we can reclaim the lost or abandoned parts of our inner beings, and similarly appreciate and help others bring forth those abandoned, vulnerable parts of themselves. In a very real way, we can, like Beauty, through our compassion transform into princes the Beasts of our own lives.

6. COOPERATION

When pain strikes we often ask the wrong questions, such as, Why me? The right questions are, What can I learn from this? What can I do about it? What can I accomplish in spite of it?

Norman Vincent Peale

There is a wonderful saying: "Don't push the river." It is a reminder of how much of our lives we spend "swimming against the current," getting nowhere, only to discover that our true success and inner peace are found when we respect the river and go with the current. As you use your observation and compassion to perceive opportunities for cooperation, you will experience a profound sense of freedom. Cooperation empowers us, allowing us to look beyond being victims of circumstances or slaves to our own illnesses.

Back in 1981, Michael and I went on a white water rafting trip on the Cheet River in West Virginia. I wanted to prove to myself that even with multiple sclerosis I could be courageous and daring, doing whatever I wanted to do. We came to an area in the river appropriately named Killer Rapids. Crashing through the churning waters, the boat bucked and heaved, violently thrown this way and that by the tremendous power of the river.

Suddenly, I was thrown from the safety of the boat into the rushing waters, hitting my head on a rock and breaking my nose. The force of the river pulled me under, and a part of me just let go, *cooperating*, flowing with the river, not resisting it. I have never known such peace. I heard choral music sung by a melodic choir; I smelled the sweet fragrance of frangipani flowers; I saw flashes of purple and white light; I heard a clear voice saying, "Do not fear; you are safe. I will always be with you."

At that moment, I remember making a promise to myself, that no matter what, I would find this peaceful place again, this inner place of loving. It was a place of total cooperation, accepting what was in front of me, flowing with the water, not resisting, and not fearing what at the moment seemed like imminent death.

The greatest discovery of my generation is that a human being can alter his life by altering his attitudes of mind.

William James

So many times, when I find myself playing the victim and fighting my illness, I try to remind myself of that white water experience. Serious illness is like the river. It can come at us with a relentless power that can fill us with fear and despair. But if we have developed these first five keys of living successfully with illness—Honesty, Acceptance, Patience, Observation, and Compassion—we can *find the place of peace where we can cooperate, flowing with the current and discovering how to move with its power rather than fighting it.*

There is no real guarantee that the sun will come up tomorrow, but through maintaining our faith, we know it will. We *know*, and this type of faith becomes so strong nothing can shake it. Remaining in this place of calm, acceptance, patience, and observation made it possible for me to find my own way once I had been shown the Light.

Do not worry about whether or not the sun will rise.
Be prepared to enjoy it.

Anonymous

Beauty's cooperation launches both her and the Beast toward a change neither of them could have foreseen when she stops resisting the life she has been swept into against her own will. Each day her cooperation brings her closer to the Beast and closer to the truth within her own heart. When he falls ill, compassion and cooperation move her to respond to the reality of the illness and to his vulnerability. By flowing with the current, which might have terrified others, both of them open up to their greatest strengths and move toward that oneness of consciousness called God.

Prayer

I asked God for strength that I might achieve,
I was made weak, that I might learn humbly to obey.

I asked for health, that I might do greater things,
I was given infirmity, that I might do better things.

I asked for riches, that I might be happy,
I was given poverty, that I might be wise.

I asked for power, that I might have the praise of men,
I was given weakness, that I might feel the need of God.

I asked for all things, that I might enjoy life,
I was given life, that I might enjoy all things.

I got nothing I asked for—
but everything I had hoped for.

Almost despite myself,
my unspoken prayers were answered.

I am among all men,
Most richly blessed.

Unknown Confederate soldier

7. Loyalty

This above all: to thine own self be true,
And it must follow, as the night the day,
Thou canst not then be false to any man.

William Shakespeare

Webster's New American Dictionary defines loyalty as "manifesting fidelity; faithful; constant in devotion or regard." At its deepest level, loyalty means being true to yourself, aided by the guidance of the six previous steps in the process for change we're exploring here. The power to change, to live one's life completely and fully, regardless of health issues you may be facing, is the pinnacle of loyalty as we use the term here. In this context, loyalty is synonymous with fidelity, faithfulness, devotion and regard for life itself and for the spiritual reality that all life mirrors. Your devotion and loyalty keep you moving forward. Be loyal to faithfully finding new truths and to creating and building on those areas of truth. Then look to your Seven Keys for Personal Change and to what you have learned.

On December 2, 1990, Michael and I were guests at the meeting of the General Assembly of the United Nations, honoring Peace Prayer Day, a celebration dedicated to the children of the earth. It was a very special day for me. After twenty-five years of peace advocacy, I now found myself sitting in a room surrounded by hundreds of people from nearly all nations. As I looked around, I felt a deep bonding with every human being; this clearly was a place where we all joined as one, loyal to one cause, despite differences in nationality, personal identity, race, color, or creed. Here was a place where we shared our loving devotion in ways that allowed us to experience each others' Light, transcending virtually all the more individualized ways we measure our own and each others' worth in everyday life.

Standing up within myself, fully in support of myself and the Spirit expressed through me, I recognized the true meaning of loyalty. My electric scooter, upon which I am dependent to move about, the tremor in my left hand, my *disability* were all forgotten. I saw and experienced only the perfection that exists beyond all that, the perfection of the spiritual source from which we all come and of which we are all expressions.

In *Beauty and the Beast,* we see both main characters dedicated throughout their lives to their versions of the Seven Keys for Personal Change: Honesty, Acceptance, Patience, Observation, Compassion, Cooperation, and Loyalty. Though they seemed to be following separate paths, in the end of the story they arrive together at the same destination, realizing the truth of the Spirit that lives beyond surface appearances or their own judgments of each other. The act of forgiveness is the healing that harmoniously links these keys together.

LIVING YOUR DREAM

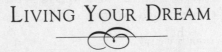

All of our dreams can come true if we have the courage to pursue them.

Walt Disney

I remember when, a few years ago, the makers of Crayola announced they were now going to be producing crayons with "multicultural" skin tones. "To prepare students to become players in a global world, educators must teach students to understand and appreciate different cultures," said Binney & Smith, explaining the reason for their new product. The child in me remembered looking through her crayon box and finding only one marked "flesh"—a pale pinkish color that never quite worked for her. We are burnt sienna. We are apricot. We are mahogany. We are peach. We are olive. We are ablebodied and physically challenged, healthy and ill. We are of all colors, shapes, sizes, and circumstances. But when we fully grasp the meaning of loyalty, through practicing the Seven Keys, we are no longer imprisoned by our perception of our separateness. Something inside of us says, "I want to be of service. I want to help. How can I?" And the answer may come forward very quietly in the silence. To be able to serve is a great blessing. We can be any color, or all colors, and recognize our common bond in the spiritual source from which we all come.

EXPRESSIONS OF LOYALTY

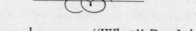

You see things; and you say, "Why?" But I dream things that never were; and I say, "Why not?"

George Bernard Shaw

Loyalty is expressed in an infinite number of ways, large and small, every moment of our lives. It is expressed each time we commit ourselves fully to any thought or act, using the seven principles we've outlined here to bring our full aliveness to the moment. This loyalty may be expressed and experienced:

- With each breath we take
- By getting up each time we fall
- By determining to go on—no matter what!
- By creating a support network
- By appreciating the positive stepping stones of life's experience
- By trusting our own inner resources
- By listening to our inner direction

- By loving ourselves enough to ask for support
- By seeking spiritual growth as the real healing
- By becoming more attuned to the Light
- By going forward and asking to be of service

Looking at my life through this vision of loyalty, which embodies all seven principles for change, I see that my hand is still in tremor. My legs are still rigid in the brisk autumn air. I still require my scooter to get around. But I am grateful for my life. Once again, I am reminded of my true identity, beyond all the surface judgments I might make about my discomfort and the more obvious restrictions of living with multiple sclerosis. Once again, I am reminded of the power in that simple lesson of reminding ourselves that we have a choice between seeing our glass as half empty or seeing it as half full.

Life Skill #14

If you can observe this process—if you do not judge or try to change anything that you observe—then your real feelings will begin to surface. By simply allowing your feelings to express themselves, without rejecting or trying to change them in any way, you will discover the true cause of your upset. This recognition will soften the intensity of these feelings, and eventually they will just go away.

ACTIVATING THE SEVEN KEYS IN YOUR LIFE

Just trust yourself, then you will know how to live.

Johann Wolfgang von Goethe

As we close this chapter, you might find it helpful to go through the Seven Keys for Personal Change and reflect on ways you have experienced them in your own life and how you might apply them in your life today. Here are some guidelines that you may find useful.

1. HONESTY

Past experience: Think of a time in your past when you really dug in your heels and resisted or denied a particular situation. Recall how you felt while you were resisting, then how you felt when you were perfectly honest with yourself and let in that reality. This recollection could be as mundane as trying a new food that you at first thought you'd hate, to something as life-altering as coming out of denial and learning to be honest about a problem you or a loved one was facing.

Present experience: Think of a situation in your present life where you find you are resisting the truth. Ask yourself what you might do and how it would feel to honestly face that situation and move forward with it.

2. ACCEPTANCE

Past experience: Think of a time in your past when you learned to accept a difficult situation by letting go of the initial perception you had of it. Remember how you felt prior to letting go of your perception, then how you felt afterward.

Present experience: Pause, relax, and go deeply into yourself for a moment. Try to get in touch with an area where you are experiencing considerable resistance. For just a moment, let go of the perception that is causing you to resist the truth. See how it feels to let go, even if it is just for a few seconds.

3. PATIENCE

Past experience: As you think back over your life, you may be able to recognize that the actions you have taken could be divided into two groups: those you took based on pretty immediate impressions or instant gratifications and actions you took only after considerable reflection. The latter are those in which patience played an important role, allowing us to perhaps discover a way of looking at the world that was not limited to our immediate perceptions. Take a moment to note and perhaps acknowledge the role patience played in that situation—what made it difficult at the time, what helped you through it, and any benefits you realized from exercising your patience.

Present experience: Focus for a moment on the present. Take the time to get in touch with any feelings of agitation or urgency or restlessness you might be feeling. In what way are these feelings attached to a perception you are holding in your mind? And in what ways might you take a more wait-and-see approach, investing less in your perception and more in allowing the present to effortlessly unfold and reveal itself to you in its own way?

Silence is healing for all ailments.

Hebrew proverb

---

4. OBSERVATION

Past experience: Most of the time, we look at the world through the filters of our own perceptual minds. As a result, we find in the external world only what our inner perceptions will allow us to find. However, we have all had experiences when the unexpected occurred—when we suddenly noticed something that we *didn't know was there.* For example, while driving a road we have driven many times in the past, we come upon a beautiful view that we had never noticed before. Or we discover we have a special knack or skill that we never thought we had. Usually, this happens when we drop our perceptual filters, either deliberately or spontaneously, and leave an opening for a new experience. Take the time to note any experiences such as these in your past and perhaps even retrace how the key of observation worked, dropping your preconceptions long enough for you to let in the unexpected and the beauty of the moment.

Present experience: Is there a situation in your life where you might benefit from taking the position of a more detached observer, being aware of what's occurring without getting actively involved? If you sense that there is, take the position of the observer starting right now. In the beginning, you may be able to do it only for a second or two. But with regular practice, you'll find your skill as an observer getting stronger and stronger.

5. Compassion

Forgiveness is the key to action and freedom.

Hannah Arendt

Past experience: True compassion begins with ourselves. Think of a time in your past when instead of judging yourself for your behavior or an action you had once felt was a weakness or a negative attribute, you became more understanding, forgiving, and compassionate. At such moments, we usually feel more loving and caring toward ourselves. In turn, as we become more understanding and loving toward ourselves, we extend these same ways of relating toward others. Try to recall what you felt in these relationships.

Present experience: Stop and reflect for a moment on ways that you are judging yourself or others harshly at this time. For just a moment, forgive yourself for your judgments and seek a more caring approach to understanding. Let love replace your judgments, letting go of any past grievance or guilts that might be involved.

6. Cooperation

Past experience: Particularly when we are faced with "bad news," we react with resistance or even disgust. We begin to *push the river*, fighting the current instead of working with it. Sometimes this comes out as resistance to other people or as defensiveness about something we don't want to hear. Recall turning points in your life when you stopped resisting or being defensive, when you stopped pushing the river and started working with the situation or people around you. Note how you felt at this time and any benefits you gained after successfully negotiating this turning point.

Present experience: Identify an area in your life where you are presently pushing the river, resisting, or being defensive. For only a moment, stop and imagine ways that you might cooperate with that situation. For a moment, envision ways your life might actually improve through cooperation. Note any internal self-talk that is urging you to either go forward and cooperate or resist. Be reminded here that you are not required to cooperate or to resist; you are simply noting what you are experiencing when you imagine yourself doing one or the other. Notice if you are experiencing more peace inside when you cooperate with life the *way it is.*

7. LOYALTY

*One can never consent to creep when one feels an
impulse to soar.*

Helen Keller

Past experience: When we put all the above keys together, we experience our lives in ways that are characteristically fuller and richer than perhaps they are most of the time. This is true whether we have an illness or not. And the lesson here is that when we apply the Seven Keys earnestly and sincerely, illness does not prevent us from enjoying our lives to the fullest. The joy of mastery within you sustains you here as it takes you higher, deeper, and into even greater fulfillment.

You may, at this time, find it helpful to recall moments in your past when you experienced your life this way. It may have occurred in your job when, after working very hard over a period of time to complete a specific task, you not only completed it but felt unusually fulfilled, knowing that you accomplished what you did through the kind of loyalty we have been exploring here. You may have had a similar kind of experience as the result of a more personal dedicated effort, ranging from courageously moving your arms and legs that have been motionless for some time to presenting a speech in a public situation. All of these experiences can help put you in touch with the quality of life open to you through the Seven Keys.

Present experience: Whether you are well or ill, ablebodied or physically challenged, you can enjoy the quality of life that we have been examining in this chapter. The exercises you have already completed take you to the threshold where this becomes possible. At this point, focus on just one small area in your life where you might apply all Seven Principles. This might be in an important relationship with a friend or relative. It might be in a creative or athletic endeavor in physical therapy. Or it might be in learning a new skill, finishing a jigsaw puzzle, writing a letter to a friend, cooking some new dishes, or fixing up the house.

LOOKING AHEAD

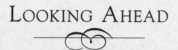

In the next chapter, "Who We Become," we'll be turning our attention to the meaning of relationships and how the life skills we've been exploring throughout this book can be employed in that area of our lives. When you love, you don't look at anything as being a burden or a sacrifice. Anyone who has learned to live successfully with an illness knows the importance of creating truly quality relationships, ones that are validating, healing, supportive, and loving. As you go on to this next chapter, you will find that everything you've read in the previous chapters, and particularly the one you've just finished, comes into sharp focus here.

As you turn to the next chapter, you may wish to take a moment to glance back over the material we've covered so far. Just flipping through the pages of this book, or perhaps looking back over entries you've made in your journal, will be helpful as you move ahead on this upward path.

You have to leave the city of your comfort and go into the wilderness of your intuition. What you'll discover will be wonderful. What you'll discover will be yourself.

Alan Alda

5

Who We Become: Building Healing Relationships That Matter

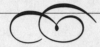

Independence? That's middle-class blasphemy.
We are all dependent on one another—
every soul of us on earth.

George Bernard Shaw

As we've discussed throughout this book, serious illness does have a way of exaggerating our illusions about being different from others, of being special or unworthy, and of ultimately being separate and alone. When we are feeling this way, life can indeed appear quite unmanageable and we can feel completely overwhelmed; after all, if we see ourselves as alone, we are also laboring under the illusion that there is nobody to help us, that we must carry our load alone. To know that these feelings are illusions, not truths, can be liberating, particularly if we can get some insight into their source and what we might do to move beyond them; that is what this chapter is about.

As to the source of our illusions, you can be quite assured that if you grew up in the United States or in any part of the world that is strongly influenced by our beliefs, you've probably inherited at least a small portion of the "rugged individualist" syndrome, the idea that our self-worth is measured by our independence, "beholden to nobody." To some degree, we all mirror what some consider to be our national neurosis—the illusion that we are nothing if we can't *go it alone*. Since most of us do embrace the spirit of the rugged individualist, it can be comforting to know that the aloneness we feel is not a product of illness so much as it is a product of perceptions associated with this limited view of life.

As George Bernard Shaw and many other writers have pointed out over the millennia, the illusion that we are independent and alone is nothing but that: an illusion. What we can accomplish always depends not only on our individual capacities and inner resources but on different types of support networks all around us. We need go no further than the example of this book to see this principle at work. A book such as you now hold in your hands would not be possible without editors, other writers and teachers, and a whole raft of support people from the publishing community —from people carrying mail back and forth, to editors, to clerks in the Library of Congress, to book designers, printers, truckers, booksellers, and book buyers—the list could go on and on!

When we study other cultures, particularly the cultures of early indigenous peoples, we discover a much deeper appreciation for the infinite ways in which we are all dependent on support from sources outside us. The Lakota, for example, have a short prayer that says "We are all One," which they repeat in virtually all of their ceremonies. It is a way of reminding the Lakota people of how their lives are interwoven not only with the people around them but with the whole fabric of the natural world. "We are all One" is a reminder that no life could survive on this planet without an endless circle of support.

In so many ways, a key to our healing—be it physical, mental, emotional, or spiritual—is found in the feelings of being connected, validated, and trusted. It is found in how we express the same feelings toward others, in giving and receiving support in a variety of ways. From some people we learn the best ways to work with medical professionals who can help us. From others we learn how to better work within systems or organizations, such as the medical system, the social service system, the community at large. Through still other individuals or groups we find role models who give us new hope or courage, or we discover new sources of motivation that allow us to take risks. We have people in our lives who nurture us when we are in crisis or who help us get back on our feet after a crippling challenge.

While it feels good to know that we are loved and supported by others, these feelings are not just a matter of sentiment. It is now known that our relationships with others can have a direct effect on the human body's inborn self-healing mechanisms. This is by no means an idle claim. Writing in 1990 in the *Lancet*, the highly esteemed medical journal, Dr. Dean Ornish stated, "The subjective experience of feeling consciously connected with others and with our environment (or that which is larger than ourselves) has been found to promote physical and mental health, or well-being."

WHAT SUPPORT NETWORKS MAY INCLUDE

At the heart of each of us, whatever our imperfections, there exists a silent pulse of perfect rhythm, a complex of wave forms and resonances, which is absolutely individual and unique, and yet which connects us to everything in the universe.

George Leonard

Each human's needs cover a very wide range, and none of us can say that all our needs can ever be met by a single person or group, much less that we can meet all our needs alone. Our support network may include any or all of the following:

Intimates: Our spouses, children, siblings, parents, and extended family members, who provide deep emotional support and the *blood bonds* that help us to feel part of something larger than ourselves.

Friends: People outside our families, with whom we share special interests or values, people who are likeminded or with whom we have heart connections that we find give us strength, support, and a sense of self-worth.

Co-workers: These can be individuals or groups (professional associations, labor unions, and so on) who provide us with information and support associated with our work.

Service people: Baby-sitters, carpenters, window washers, plumbers, housekeepers, cable TV installers, pest exterminators, secretarial workers, taxi drivers, and so forth.

Professionals: Counselors, medical advisers, business associates, teachers, physicians, pharmacists, clergy, therapists, and so on.

It is important to note here, of course, that we are ourselves members of similar support networks for others. Each of us belongs to at least two of these support groups.

ACTS OF KINDNESS

Our chief want in life is somebody who will make us do what we can.

Ralph Waldo Emerson

As you become more aware of the function of support networks in your life, it can be useful to take the time to actually note some of the human needs that we can expect to be satisfied, in whole or in part, by others. Take the time to think about each of the following and perhaps record your responses in your journal.

1. To whom do you turn for laughter, closeness, and a sense of intimacy?

2. Who is (are) your best supporter(s) when you are faced with a difficult challenge?

3. With whom do you share commitments to pursue your dreams?

4. To whom do you turn when you wish to be motivated to your next levels of learning and self-mastery?

5. To whom do you turn for empowerment and visions of personal success?

6. With whom do you share spiritual issues in your life?

7. Who do you call when you want to go shopping for new clothes or a special item?

8. Who assists you on a daily basis?

9. Who in your life reminds you of self-responsibility and consciousness growth?

10. Who encourages or supports you to deeper levels of involvement and creativity?

11. Who do you seek out for referrals or suggestions?

12. Whose company provides you with relaxed, easy, safe, high-quality companionship?

13. To whom do you turn when you are hurting?

14. Where do you go when you want to be part of a supportive learning environment?

15. With whom do you discuss politics, gender and racial issues, world events?

BUILDING OUR SUPPORT NETWORKS

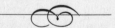

Most of us go through life not knowing what we want,
but feeling darned sure this isn't it.

Anonymous

So often when we have an illness, our self-judgments create separation in ways that can be as perplexing as they are devastating. Out of our own sense of unworthiness, we may feel, say, or do things that actually make it quite impossible for other people to be part of our lives. I recently had an experience that illustrated this in a way that is not at all uncommon.

My friend Fran, a woman in her seventies, called me on the

phone and was complaining that because her cousin had failed to give her a ride, she had been unable to attend a friend's birthday party. She said, "When I see her next time, I'm really going to let her have it!"

"Was she supposed to pick you up?" I asked.

"Of course she was," Fran replied. "She knows I don't drive."

"Did you call and ask her for a ride?"

"No. I shouldn't have to. She should know I need her help. She picked me up once before."

"Which was when?" I asked.

"Oh, I don't know," Fran snapped. "Maybe three or four years ago."

I happened to know that the cousin who "should have" picked her up thought the world of Fran. A simple phone call, and I am certain she would have been overjoyed to help out. When I told Fran this, she became quite agitated, claiming that if her cousin really cared for her she would have called and offered a ride.

Life Skill #15

Whether your giving exhausts or invigorates you will depend on your attitude. We get into all kinds of traps when we communicate with specific expectations. Perhaps you have said, "I love you" with the unconscious expectation of hearing "I love you" back. If it didn't come, you may have felt that something was wrong. That's not communication; that's fishing. To say "I feel wonderful when you say *I love you.* I wish you would say it more" is a clear message, letting the other person know both how you are feeling and what you'd like from them.

My conversation with Fran was a reminder to me of how our own perceptions can embitter and entrap us, making us feel even more isolated and alone than we already are. What is it that prevents us from asking for help, that so often results in our judging others for being uncaring because they can't *read our minds?* The reasons are as varied as our own tastes, ranging from feeling too proud or frightened to feeling embarrassed or obligated to others. We feel deficient, helpless, unlovable, or needy. And instead of checking in with other people to find out what they are really feeling, we project our own judgments of ourselves onto them. We literally turn potential friends and supporters into enemies. The process of projecting our thoughts and feelings onto others isn't part of being ill, and it isn't abnormal in any way. On the contrary, as we've discussed in previous chapters, we normally *make sense of the world* through our projections, then our interpretations. When we can take full responsibility for this very human process, however, we put ourselves in the position of being able to choose: are we going to project our perception of unworthiness onto others, or are we going to project our love? Depending on which we choose, we will either enjoy support or deepen our sense of isolation.

In my own life, I know that I would probably not have looked quite so closely at my own projections, and thus would never have enjoyed the sense of freedom I have today, had it not been for my illness. As a friend once related to me in a letter, "In normal, everyday life, our projections are usually good enough. We get by, hardly noticing that we don't give others much of a chance to let us know who they really are. We cover up our sense of isolation and loneliness by staying busy, distracting ourselves by whatever means we can find. Television and excessive sleep are examples. But when we are ill, we start seeing life as if through a very big magnifying glass. It gets harder and harder to deceive ourselves. Then it can literally become a life and death matter to examine our projections very carefully."

Learning to look at our projections, to better understand how they affect the quality of our lives, and how we might manage them so that we can live more fully, is perhaps one of the greatest gifts we can give ourselves, illness or not. But how do we do this?

We begin by looking upon our experiences of the outer world as metaphorical feedback mechanisms that mirror our projections back to us and ask us to look at ourselves in a new way. The payoff is that we expand our ability to enjoy and reap the benefits of our relationships in ways that might otherwise be quite impossible. As we begin moving beyond our projections, our hearts literally open up.

Sometimes what we see isn't all that pleasant. We discover in the reflections that the outer world mirrors back to us aspects of ourselves that we'd just as soon keep hidden. As the French artist and writer Jean Cocteau once remarked, partly in jest, "Mirrors should reflect a little before throwing back images." In other words, as we remember my conversation with my friend Fran, once we do start looking at our projections to the outer world as mirroring back aspects of ourselves, we discover that the world offers some frank and brutally honest revelations. Very often, I find, I wouldn't be willing to be so honestly introspective with myself if I had no health problems or if learning to live successfully with illness wasn't the top priority in my life.

Recently, I was challenged with an experience that offers an excellent example of what I'm describing here. I had gotten a referral to a neurologist I'd never met before, in the process of trying to find out more about the uncontrollable tremor in my left hand. As I entered, his receptionist was extremely brusque and snappish, which immediately put me off. After examining me, the doctor scribbled things down in my chart and, without even looking up to acknowledge me, said something to the effect that the shaking was the result of a lesion in the upper motor region on the right side of my brain.

"It's classic MS," he stated arrogantly, "an *intention tremor*."

Hundreds of unanswered questions were flowing through my mind. *Were there any non-chemical treatments that might help? What exactly was going on with the unwelcome intruder? Was there anything I could do, any route I might pursue, that could help reduce the tremor?* I wanted alternatives, recommendations, potential solutions, guidance, a glimmer of hope—some sense that my life somehow mattered.

I felt my anger and resentment growing, directed toward this cool, seemingly uninterested and arrogant physician. I observed myself resenting his cool, impenetrable manner. As you read this, you will probably agree that the physician should have been more compassionate and responsive. And certainly a case could be made for that. But clinging to these judgments, however "justified" they might be, doesn't get us much more than more pain.

Instead of clinging to my judgments about him, and insisting they were the only truth, I began to ask myself what the things I was feeling might teach me about myself. I asked how much of the frustration I was feeling toward the doctor came from my frustration with this new symptom that I was apparently going to have to accept about myself. Clearly, this was an aspect of the experience I couldn't deny.

And what about his arrogance? I asked. Notwithstanding the fact that it is never an attractive trait, I also recognized that his behavior mirrored my own arrogance. I knew from past experience that I adopted an arrogant posture as a way to distance myself from other people when I was feeling fearful and unworthy. The trouble was that it always made matters worse, creating illusions of separation that made me feel even more afraid and small.

Notice that I am not denying that this physician really did appear to be arrogant in his behavior or that I was projecting my frustration with my tremor into the relationship between us. But the top priority for me was how the experience was a useful mirror to me. As soon as I could see and accept my part in the discomfort I was feeling, I could begin to forgive myself for the judgments I was making about the whole situation. That very act of judgment, I knew, was the source of my sense of separation, fear, and aloneness. And as soon as I was able to forgive myself for judging the physician, I began to feel better—not, I think, because I was letting him off the hook but because I was forgiving myself for my judgments. The judgments against myself, incidentally, were far more damaging than the tremor in my left hand.

In all these mirroring experiences, I remember the following little exercise given to me by my good friend Mary. It allows me to see the various people in my life in the light of being worthy and loving members of my support network.

I forgive myself for judging my feelings.
I forgive myself for judging myself as unworthy.
I forgive myself for judging myself as I am remembering who
    I am:
I am a radiant being, filled with Light and loving.

To take responsibility for our own consciousness in this way is a relatively easy process, and one that can open up the world to us in ways that are almost unimaginable. At the core of it is *judgment*— judgment that begins with our own judgments about ourselves. The moment we begin forgiving ourselves for judging ourselves, we discover how full our lives can be. Our own humanness, and the humanness of everyone around us, rushes in and literally fills our hearts. In the process, our support networks grow, and almost miraculously the quality of these relationships improves.

The act of judgment is like a heavy iron door slamming shut. Once shut, we are imprisoned behind the bars of our own perceptions and beliefs. So often, our judgments come quickly and automatically—and usually appear to be fully "justified" by something we or another person has done or has failed to do. Certainly there's no denying that we all do things that are reproachable, but if we can see no further than this, our judgments only end up limiting and crippling us.

The minute I was able to forgive myself for judging my feelings triggered by the physician's brusque and arrogant treatment, our relationship changed. I began to see this neurologist as a resource, though he was not able to tell me what I wanted to hear. We actually parted company on a very friendly note and I went away feeling better about myself, far closer to accepting the reality of this new tremor.

Life Skill #16

In order to communicate, you must first accept yourself as you are, and as good enough just as you are. Every human being—*every person alive*—is truly a valuable, worthwhile being. Remind yourself of that, particularly during emotional times when you may be feeling frustrated, fearful, and judgmental. Remind yourself that the person to whom you are talking is a valuable, worthwhile human being (even if he or she isn't behaving the way you might wish).

LEARNING TO SEE OTHERS AS MIRRORS

But before I look out . . . let me first gaze within myself.

Rainer Maria Rilke

It definitely takes practice to make the kind of shift in perception that I've just described. The following eight questions can be helpful guides as you begin applying these principles in your own life.

1. What is it about others' behavior that most often triggers your judgments about them?

EXAMPLE:
I can't stand people who yell at their children and put them down.

2. What do you tell yourself about people who do this?

EXAMPLE:
I judge them as ignorant, selfish, and fearful.

3. What is your judgment of how they *should* act?

EXAMPLE:
They should learn to be kind and loving, disagreeing with their kids without being disagreeable.

4. What would you like to do about their behavior?

EXAMPLE:
I vacillate between telling myself I should accept their behavior and love them anyway, or telling them that their behavior really bothers me and I'd like them to treat their kids better.

5. What can you do *within yourself* to resolve these judgments against others?

EXAMPLE:
I can forgive myself for judging them, recognizing that in my judgments I am somehow attacking something in myself. I can also be reminded that my standards of behavior may not always be appropriate for others.

6. What lesson does this mirror of behavior offer you?

EXAMPLE:
It reminds me to be more forgiving within myself as I learn more about acceptance for who I am.

7. How can you apply these lessons?

EXAMPLE:
I can begin to heal hurtful memories from my own childhood.
I can be gentler with myself, knowing that what triggers my
judgment of critical parents is perhaps my own inner parent
who is so critical toward my own inner child. Knowing that
the behavior I criticize in others might be coming from a
similar place, I find myself having more compassion for both of
us—a process that seems to be deeply satisfying, healing the
child in everyone concerned.

8. In what ways can you bring these new understandings into
your relationships with the people you have been judging?

EXAMPLE:
I can begin by acknowledging my judgments the moment I
make them, then forgive myself for judging and be reminded
of this lesson. I do not yet know where this will lead me except
that I will then be more open and loving, able to be more
responsive to whatever opportunities arise for my healing.

PERCEPTION = INTERPRETATION

The lover is looking in a mirror in which
he is beholding his Self.

Plato

As we reflect on this process of projection, it's important to remember that it is not just negativity that we project on to others or find
mirrored in their behavior. It is also our loving and caring, our
generosity, loyalty, and humor. When we are forgiving and loving
with ourselves, we invariably project that to others, and they, in
feeling it, perhaps take it in, healing their own self-judgments and
giving back exactly what we have given. Nearly all projections, I
believe, move in a circle, a circle that takes in everyone around us.
This very well may be one of the most important discoveries we
will make about creating our support networks and making the
relationships we establish within them fulfilling for everyone concerned.

KNOWING WHAT YOU WANT

You've got to be very careful if you don't know where you are going, because you might not get there.

Yogi Berra

Every human being, ill or well, has a great variety of needs that involve other people's help. This can include obvious basic needs, such as food, shelter, or wanting a ride somewhere, as well as less obvious and more intimate needs, such as emotional and spiritual support. Some of these needs are pretty straightforward and easy for us to communicate and have met. Others are linked up with strong emotional charges that make them difficult for us to state. For example, ordering a meal in a restaurant is usually a simple transaction, with very little ambiguity or hidden emotional content; getting a stranger to help you in the bathroom, however, can be quite another matter.

Wherever we have a strong emotion associated with asking for what we want, there's a high potential for us to communicate our ambivalence or fear. One of the dangers in this is that we push people away rather than getting our needs met. We don't get what we want because we are afraid to ask. We think, "They won't have the time"; "I shouldn't trouble them"; "They should know—I shouldn't have to ask"; "I don't know them well enough." Because of these assumptions, we may never even risk enough to test our beliefs. And the lesson I've learned is that when we stay emotionally in touch with our needs, and express them clearly, without all the overlays of feeling unworthy or projecting our distrust to others, support grows and expands.

It takes courage to push yourself to places that you have never been before . . . to test your limits . . . to break through barriers.

Anonymous

If there is nothing else my illness has taught me, it is that if we are to live successfully with illness, it's important to understand our projections. Trapped momentarily by our fear, our self-judgments, and our sense of unworthiness, we may communicate some pretty confusing messages. For example, had my friend Fran been able to go through the process of looking at what the world was mirroring back to her, she might have been able to see that it was she, not her cousin, who was creating her isolation. Without knowing it, Fran herself made certain that she would be left at home, unable to attend her friend's party.

Life Skill #17

One way to demonstrate honesty with another is to keep all communication clear in the moment it is happening. If somebody tells you something you don't understand, or if you feel misunderstood, or if you feel you are not being heard, tell the person about it. Don't wait until tomorrow. Trust in the relationship enough to speak honestly in every moment.

For whatever reasons, it has never been easy for me to ask for what I wanted, and I have always been resistant to asking other people for support. Throughout the early part of my life, I felt that if I should ever stand up for myself, others might think of me as pushy, conceited, self-centered, determined, being on a high-horse, assertive, egotistical, self-righteous, self-absorbed, selfish, or vain. In my youth, I was so self-conscious about these qualities that I often found myself somewhat embarrassed about my last name—Noble.

---

*I bid him look into the lives of men as though into a mirror,
and from others to take an example for himself.*

Terence

Illness challenged me to move beyond my I'll-do-it-all-myself stance in life, to reach out, be authentic, forgive myself for my judgments that I wasn't worthy of asking for other people's support, or that I could not trust others to give me what I wanted. It has not always been easy to move beyond these self-judgments, but in doing so I discovered how much I limited myself and how rich life could be when I released myself from that prison.

I have begun to understand that in all support relationships there is an important exchange of energy, from one person to another and back again, moving in a circle. And this happens in all relationships, whether they are long-term, as in the case of a lifelong friend or family member, or only fleeting, as with the young woman who helped me in the ladies room. Because of this movement of energy between us, every relationship has the potential for being support-ive, uplifting our spirits. Even stopping to give a stranger directions, and really taking the time to be truly helpful to him or her, can be nurturing for both of us. By the same token, we may use the same powerful exchange of energy to create relationships that nurture and support us in more intimate ways.

Life Skill #18

As you learn to open your heart to yourself, you will find yourself opening your heart to others. Serving with an open heart is what nourishes and fulfills both the giver and the receiver.

Over the past seven years, I have formed a close alliance with three other people. Though they are not part of my regular circle of social friends, we are following a similar path together, centered on the leadership and guidance of Spirit. Our silent contract is to empower and support ourselves and one another unconditionally as we look at what the mirror of life is presenting us. We speak regularly on the telephone, and meet twice a month as a group. We focus our atten-tion on our victories—"I'm so proud about . . ." or "I want to really acknowledge myself for . . ."—but neither do we ignore our defeats: "I feel lost. I can't find my way out of this" or "What gives me hope is . . ."

The support and acknowledgment we give and receive take place in a nonjudgmental atmosphere, one of unconditional caring, in the

service of ourselves and one another. Our mission is to enjoy ourselves as we discover and share the beauty and majesty of our true
spiritual essence.

SHARING OUR CRAYONS

You have to know what you want to get.

Gertrude Stein

The challenge of illness takes me back to my basic elementary
education. It teaches me to share my crayons and ask for what I
want.

During the past holiday season, Michael and I had our annual
neighborhood block party. It was bitterly cold, and my legs and
lower back were rigid and painful to the touch. We were expecting
sixty people to attend the party, and though I was unable to participate in the preparations I was determined not to cancel this event.
It was my favorite time of the year and I looked forward to it with
great pleasure.

In earlier years, I think I would have canceled rather than ask
other people for help. But over the previous year, I had learned to
value and honor my relationships in a new way. I had learned to be
very clear about asking for what I want, dissolving old feelings that
I need to do everything for myself. I had begun to be perhaps a little
more peaceful with that part of me that imposed perfectionistic,
artistic standards on everyone around me. I had learned of pleasures
beyond this—for example, the very special pleasure of feeling the
generosity of giving and receiving unconditionally, realizing that
the real value of living is found in the human exchanges we share.

I contacted friends and neighbors and communicated exactly
what I wanted. Gail designed invitations. Gloria put them in our
neighbors' mailboxes. Afterward, she called me up to say how much
she'd enjoyed the long, brisk walk in the fresh winter air. Later, she
arrived before all the other guests to decorate our house with holly
and other evergreens from our bushes.

Jim and Robin loaned us their punch bowl and we filled it with
hot apple cider. David brought in firewood and stacked it by the

fireplace. Marylee welcomed people at the door. As each guest entered, he or she brought something delicious to eat and handed it to Denis to arrange on the table.

Surprisingly, I found it easy to give up control. I let go of my need to "have things right," to do them "my way." There was a spirit of joy and giving in the air as they all took part in creating an atmosphere that truly did justice to the season. For me it was a celebration of my graduation from the I'll-do-it-all-myself school, where I'd known a sense of loneliness and fear, to the school of sharing support, where we discover our true oneness.

RECOGNIZING GOODNESS

It is one of the most beautiful compensations of this life
that no man can sincerely try to help another without
helping himself.

Ralph Waldo Emerson

Where do we start with this process of learning to ask for what we want? You might find it helpful to work with the following questions, adapted from the book *One-Minute Self-Esteem*, by Candy Semigran. Use your journal to record your thoughts and feelings.

- What is it you want that you aren't asking for now?
- What prevents you from asking for it?
- If you did ask, what's the worst that could happen?
- If you did ask, what's the best that could happen?
- Being completely honest with yourself, what do you really believe is likely to happen if you ask?
- To what extent is your sense of unworthiness or distrust determining your reluctance to ask?

Having asked yourself these questions, and thought about your replies, take just a moment to suspend your self-judgments. In this frame of mind, loving yourself unconditionally, write down exactly whom you would ask and what you would ask for. As you do so, imagine there is someone in your life who you are completely confident would be your support person. This might be a real person in the present or from the past. It could be a fictional person from a book you have read or other entertainment you have enjoyed. Or, it could be someone you have made up in your own mind. Whoever it is, his or her main qualities should be those of wanting to be helpful and enjoying the exchange when you make your request. As you do this, you may find it helpful to repeat this self-affirmation.

I AM WORTHY OF LOVING AND BEING LOVED.
I AM WORTHY OF RECEIVING LOVE.

With your ideal support person in mind, think about your own circle of friends and family members. Pick out the person who is most likely to be able to hear your request and derive some pleasure from being helpful to you. Even if you have some doubts, practice in your mind making your request known to that person, in the same way that you did with the ideal helper you imagined above.

Finally, think about ways to make this request in real life. Use the model you created when you imagined the ideal support person. Determine that you will make your real request in the same way. Then set a time and place where you will actually do it.

This simple exercise sets your intent and provides you with the guidelines for building support networks that have something to offer everyone concerned.

GIVING AND RECEIVING ARE THE SAME

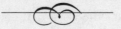

*It's not how much you do, but how much love you put
into the action.*

Mother Teresa

My two cats, Lucy and Sasha, have been wonderful teachers for me in the fine art of giving and receiving. During the day, they take turns grooming each other. Lucy receives patiently, while Sasha gives unconditionally. Then the roles are reversed, with Sasha receiving while Lucy gives unconditionally. Each appears to savor the giving as much as the receiving. What's more, when I watch them closely, I discover there is something they give even as they are receiving, which the other cat enjoys.

So often in human relationships, giving and receiving are conditional. That is, we consciously or unconsciously set up contracts: I will scratch your back as long as you scratch my back in return. Somehow the pleasure of giving is incomplete. Is it that we don't know how to take in the pleasures of giving? Or is it that we have forgotten how to receive, that in receiving we are withholding whatever magical ingredient my cats know that makes the giver happy?

Husbands and wives sometimes get into horrendous fights, ending up in the divorce courts, over the fact that one feels he or she gives more than the other. And, of course, sometimes it's true; when the giving and receiving aren't working, one person can very well feel burned out and unappreciated. But we perhaps too often jump to the conclusion that the reason we're unhappy is that we're not getting as much as we give; maybe the real problem is that we have forgotten how to enjoy unconditional giving. It is quite clear, as I watch my cats, that *each* gets great pleasure from giving. For both of them, giving and receiving are the same.

Life Skill #19

Your own personal growth is central to all the growth you provide to others. To serve others is to become more receptive and open to yourself. Each time you assist another, you are renewed and strengthened. In such circumstances, giving is also receiving. Keep these ideas in mind the next time you have the opportunity to help someone.

This is not to say there can't be imbalances. When the energy of giving and receiving flows smoothly, we feel loved and supported. Our lives seem abundant and full. When the energy is uneven, we may feel angry, frustrated, and disappointed. Within each of us, we must know how to find pleasure in both giving and receiving.

As a person with illness, I am always reminding myself that I *do* have something to give. Because I am so often on the receiving end,

I need to be alert to the ways I make a positive difference in the lives of those who support and comfort me. Most people who have an illness are in a position where it is easy for an imbalance in giving and receiving to exist. And very few people ever stop to realize that there is a particular sense of scarcity we encounter when we are deprived of the experience of giving.

THE NEED TO GIVE

All you have shall someday be given;
Therefore, give now,
that the season of giving may be yours.

Kahlil Gibran

When we are dependent on others to help us move about, to feed us, to bathe us, and to help us in the bathroom, we may easily forget that there are many other ways that we can give besides those that require physical strength and full mobility:

- We give through caring, sharing, loving; through being a good listener when others close to us want to share their thoughts and feelings.
- We give by offering little intimacies with those we care about —offering a foot massage, a back rub, even telling a joke.
- We give from the heart by sharing our vulnerabilities and expressing our emotions, through forgiveness of ourselves and others.
- We give by discovering our own qualities and finding ways they can make a positive difference in someone else's life. These qualities might include compassion, understanding, courage, clarity, perseverance, inner strength, purpose, encouragement, inspiration, humor, enthusiasm, joy, truth, gratitude, spontaneity, thoughtfulness, appreciation, and intention.
- We give by learning the joy of giving without conditions or attachments, be it through money, wisdom, time, creativity, a special skill, our life experience, or our hearts.

May it be, O Lord,
that I seek not so much to be consoled as to console,
to be understood as to understand,
to be loved as to love,
because it is in giving oneself that one receives;
it is in forgetting oneself that one is found.

Saint Francis of Assisi

There is a special lesson in anonymous giving, one that has to do with learning the pleasure of giving without expecting to receive anything back. Here are some examples of anonymous giving:

- Anonymously send flowers to a nurse, doctor, or other medical professional who works hard but rarely receives acknowledgment.
- Leave some change in a telephone booth for the next person or a passerby to pick up.
- Anonymously pay a bill for a friend who is having financial difficulties.
- Buy two theater tickets and give them away anonymously.
- Pay the toll for the five cars behind you. Then drive on without turning around.

Be on the lookout, as you go through the day, for ways that you can add to this list, keeping both your support group and strangers in mind. Be creative and have fun!

Inasmuch as you have done it unto the least person
among you, you have done it unto me.

Jesus

As you begin giving anonymously, pay particular attention to how these *random acts of kindness* make you feel. How do you feel about being a giver? Do these anonymous gifts help you to feel more

YOU ARE NOT YOUR ILLNESS / 170

balanced energetically? What has this anonymous giving revealed about your own cycle of giving and receiving? Have you, now or in the past, given too much to others, and not received?

Life Skill #20

L istening is a sign of loving. When a person feels heard by another human being, he or she feels loved by that person. Listen to yourself. Listen to your heart. When you listen to other people, listen through your heart to their heart. When you do, you become one with them. Their sense of self-worth can be enhanced, and their sense of identity may grow stronger. They feel valuable, worthwhile, and lovable. What a gift of yourself you can give to another person!

THE WONDERFUL ART OF RECEIVING

When I watch my cats, Lucy and Sasha, it is very clear that the act of receiving and accepting is one with its own special powers. We discover that when we are the neediest, it is usually because we have not allowed ourselves to receive rather than because nobody has given. There are some important questions to ask ourselves on this subject. For example, what do you want the giver to experience as you are receiving? Joy? Gratitude? An expression of what you are feeling? Appreciation?

Devote three full days to just receiving what others give, no matter how great or small the act may seem. Give nothing in return beyond a simple thank you. In the past three days, I have noted and given particular attention to how I received the following gifts:

- Ralph, my mailman, brought the mail up the hill to my door, instead of leaving it in the mailbox down at the street.
- Chris shoveled snow from my driveway.
- Michael hugged me from behind and planted a sudden kiss on my cheek.
- A friend who dropped by complimented my new haircut.

- Michele cooked me dinner when Michael was out of town.
- My friend Lala came by to give me a massage.
- I received a holiday greeting card from an old friend.
- My friend Holly brought me apricot roses for my birthday and left them in a vase for me at my front door.

In each case, I made a point of staying in touch with how I felt as I received these gifts. In a few cases, I at first found myself resisting ("I don't deserve this" or "I'm not worthy of this attention"), then opening up my heart. As I opened up each time, my heart was filled, knowing in that instant that there was also a heartfelt pleasure in the giving for each of them—particularly when they could sense how much their gifts meant to me.

I keep my ideals, because in spite of everything, I still believe people are really good at heart.

Anne Frank

CULTIVATING YOUR GARDEN

Give some thought now to your personal network of support people. Are you limiting yourself to a small circle of people, perhaps because you are afraid to explore new avenues? When we are ill, it is a great temptation to assume that others aren't interested, don't care, or don't have the time for us. But as often as not these are our own perceptions that we are projecting onto others as a result of our sense of unworthiness or fear. Here are some ways to expand.

Extend the amount and quality of your contacts. For example, through the years I have kept up my relationships with supporters and professionals whom I worked with on The MS Initiative, as well as members, though the organization disbanded in 1989. For example, I continue to handle referrals for new clients who want counseling from former members of The MS Initiative. In November, I was asked to host a political evening for an associate I met through these contacts who is now running for Congress. Former clients of Noble Design Associates who are from the music industry helped perform in fund-raising events.

Get to know other people with situations similar to yours. Make it a point to be informed about the various resources available regarding your health situation. Talk to others who now have, or had, a condition similar to yours. Openly and honestly ask for tips and suggestions. Ask for the names of people who can help.

Become an active patient. Whenever you have the opportunity, ask your doctor or other professional person about the illness you have. If you are near a college or university that has a nursing or medical program, spend some time using the library to research your illness and its treatment. Medical books are not as difficult to read as you might think. With a medical dictionary by your side, you will find yourself quickly becoming well versed in the language used by doctors. You will learn how to ask the kinds of questions that will truly make you and your physician allies.

Introduce people to one another. Whenever opportunities arise to introduce people who can be helpful to one another, do so. The more you do this, the more others will see you as a "networking resource"; in this respect, the best networkers are the ones for whom giving and receiving are equal. And keep in mind that every new person you contact has a network of his or her own resources. By hooking these people into your contacts, you are tapping into theirs, expanding everyone's reach.

Honestly review the people in your support system. As you grow in your own right, learning how to get over the various hurdles we've described in this book, you may find that some of your own relationships are no longer supportive. You may, for example, discover that you have a relationship with another person who "gets something" out of your being weak and helpless. And you may notice, now that you are stronger, that this person is unable to be of any real support. Such relationships can pull you down, becoming destructive rather than supportive. Take a good look at this possibility and let go of those relationships that impede your own growth process.

Let people know you value their support. Remember the lessons of my cats, Sasha and Lucy: that there is pleasure in giving, just as there is pleasure in receiving. Let your support people know how much you enjoy the support they give—often.

So long as we love we serve; so long as we are loved by others, I would almost say that we are indispensable; and no man is useless while he has a friend.

Robert Louis Stevenson

SELF-NOURISHMENT

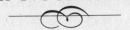

While we clearly need support from others, whether we are ill or well, we also require self-support. This refers to the loving things we do for ourselves. The three sides of this triangle I call "creating wellness" are:

- Learning to receive from others.
- Learning to give unconditionally.
- Giving to oneself.

Throughout the day, there are almost unlimited opportunities to give to ourselves. You might, for example, pause in your daily schedule to go outside and enjoy the beauty of nature, feeling the warm sun on your skin, taking a walk in a park or along a street where there are beautiful yards. You might buy yourself a small gift or take the time to read a book, go to a movie, go out to dinner with a friend, or just sit at home relaxing and enjoying a favorite video.

Each friend represents a world in us, a world possibly not born until they arrive, and it is only by this meeting that a new world is born.

Anaïs Nin

Think about specific qualities you appreciate in yourself. In the same way that you love a partner or close friend even as you recognize their shortcomings, love yourself for all that you are right now.

Yes, there may be room to grow and develop, but don't put off self-appreciation for the day you reach perfection, because—as we all know—that day will never come.

Life Skill #21

Consciously direct your inner dialogue from self-criticism to positive reinforcement, thus creating a more supportive and uplifting relationship with yourself. Developing a habit of positive self-talk takes practice and persistence. But keep at it, constantly reminding yourself of those qualities you most like in yourself.

Positive self-talk frees us from limits we consciously or unconsciously place on ourselves, and it encourages us to be more expansive in our attitudes toward ourselves. There was a time in my life when it was difficult for me to think of positive things to say about myself. At that time, in order to break that learned habit, I started a list of all the positive things I noted about myself or which other people said about me. Keeping such a list, jotting down everything that you really like about yourself or that you note others like about you, can become an extremely valuable resource and may begin a new pattern of self-support.

Use this list frequently. Look at it at the end of the day. Use the information you discover there as self-affirmations.

The world will change because of your smile . . .
To sit, to smile, to look at things and really see them—
These form the basis of peace work.

Thich Nhat Hanh

HEALTH AFFIRMATIONS

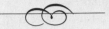

Affirmations of all kinds are powerful tools for self-support for any-one who wants to learn how to live successfully with illness. Affir-mations are strong, positive statements designed to modify negative personal beliefs. Usually, they are descriptions of a desired condi-tion; for example, the person with a negative self-image might use an affirmation to project an image of love and self-trust to himself.

The technique for designing an affirmation is a simple one: you state your desire for the future as if it has already been achieved. For example, "Each day I am getting stronger and healthier, using all my experiences, tools, and resources to learn and grow." Express the affirmation so that you are clearly the person taking the action, rather than saying, for example, "The multiple sclerosis and the chronic lower lumbar region of my spine are getting better."

It is important that you state your affirmations in a positive way. Thus, in the above example, I state that I will use "all my experi-ences, tools, and resources to learn and grow." In this way, I will not judge myself as failing on those days when my energy is low or when my hand tremor prevents me from doing my work. Rather, I will focus my attention in a positive way toward what I can learn from those more difficult days. Examples of nurturing affirmations that I use are:

All the cells in my body are now working in perfect har-mony.

My body is in balance. The energy is flowing freely and I am in a state of perfect health.

Divine love now dissolves and dissipates every negative con-dition in my mind, my body, and my circumstances.

Divine love floods my consciousness with health and every cell of my body is filled with light.

I give myself total, unconditional acceptance of myself as a loving and worthy individual.

My sense of worth cannot be measured by comparisons with others.

I feel warm and loving toward myself for I am totally worthy and perfect in my essence.

I always do the best I can with what I know and use everything to my advancement.

I let go of anything I have ever held against myself and see it dissolve into the highest light.

I stand up for my own values, opinions, and convictions and stay true to my better judgment.

I treat all problems as opportunities to grow in wisdom and love.

I am relaxed, trusting in God's plan that is unfolding for me.

I have a positively thinking mind and a perfectly healthy body.

I give myself permission to live, laugh, and love to my fullest capacity.

I am the love of Spirit.

Repeat your affirmations frequently. Each time you do this, you are building thoughts and feelings within your mind that cause you to focus on new opportunities as they arise in the constantly unfolding present of your life. The above affirmations have resulted in the following for me:

- A publishing contract for this book.
- Extensive travel with my electric scooter throughout the country on airlines that offer easy access.
- Tremors in my legs and hands not interfering with the quality of my life or my mission.
- Maintaining my spiritual life as my first priority.
- Relationships based on honesty, trust, drive, responsibility, vision, inspiration, enthusiasm, and strength.
- Using a wheelchair or walker in front of my friends without embarrassment.
- The fuller realization that *who I am is not my body but spirit.*

When writing your affirmations, keep them short, simple, and direct. Begin with phrases such as "I am" and use action verbs, usually ending in "-ing."

Charging each statement with positive energy assures that your affirmation will be fulfilled in a way that is best for everyone, including you.

PUTTING AFFIRMATIONS INTO ACTION

*"The question is," said Alice, "whether you can make
words mean so many different things."
"The question is," said Humpty Dumpty, "which is to
be master—that's all."*

Lewis Carroll

Step 1: It is a good idea to set aside certain times each day to do
your affirmations. This might be in the morning before going to
work or in the evening before going to bed.

Relax. You might even start an affirmation with a period of meditation so that you are as open and receptive as possible.

While looking into your eyes in front of a mirror, repeat your
affirmations. You should feel supported and positive as you say them.
If you don't, I recommend that you go back and restate them so that
they are uplifting and inspiring to you.

Step 2: In your mind's eye, imagine the positive result of your
affirmation already taking place. Imagine yourself enjoying the result, basking in your success.

Step 3: If you begin to feel negative or if doubts start arising in
your mind that are undermining your affirmations, don't resist them
or try to fight them off. Just observe these thoughts and feelings.
Note them as you might take note of a rainstorm, coming in, then
slowly drifting away.

For years, I struggled with negative feelings around my affirmations. When I didn't instantly get the results I wanted, I became
critical of myself; maybe I hadn't done it right, maybe it was *never*
going to work for me. When I was told by a friend that my own
negative thoughts and fears were undermining my efforts, and that
I could let these go by learning to sit back and observe them, the
whole process began to work for me. Today I can honestly say that
my affirmations have helped me modify many different ways I have
undermined myself and have helped me move forward, learning
from the challenges of my illness.

Step 4: If an affirmation doesn't seem to be truly striking an
important chord for you, or if you keep coming up with negative

thoughts and feelings around it, ask a person from your support network to help you out. Let the person read what you have written (or listen to what you have recorded, if you have used a tape recorder). Ask that person to brainstorm with you why the affirmations aren't working for you and what you might do to make them more effective. Most important, forgive yourself for judging yourself.

Step 5: It can be helpful to write your affirmations on index cards, perhaps even ones of different colors, and place them in spots where you will often see them: the refrigerator door, the dashboard of your car, the bathroom mirror, or your desk.

ULTIMATE GOALS OF SUPPORT NETWORKS

For everyone who asks receives;
He who seeks finds;
and to him who knocks,
the door will be opened.

Matthew 7 : 8

As you work on creating your affirmations, keep in mind that health is far more than the absence of illness. True health involves the whole person—body, mind, emotion, and spirit. If it can be measured at all, it is in the amount of loving energy flowing through our being. It is weighed in the *quality of life* we are able to enjoy in our relationships, regardless of the condition of our physical bodies.

Each person, every participant in our support networks, is always a mirror and a teacher for us to grow and expand. Very often it can be a great challenge to perceive our lives in this way. We get into the habit of focusing our attention on *results only*, making our first priority the physical need that is met or not met, regardless of the cost to our broader sense of emotional and spiritual well-being. It is only when we can focus on the quality of relationships we establish within our support networks that we begin to grasp what it means to live successfully with who we are—illness or not. Quality of life begins and ends with our relationships to ourselves and the world around us.

Let's keep moving on this journey to the next chapter: *"Who We Are."*

If you want to lift yourself up, lift up someone else.

Booker T. Washington

6

Who We Are

FULFILLING OUR MISSION
THROUGH SERVICE

*You cannot teach a man anything. You can only help him
discover it within himself.*

Galileo

Too often when we are ill, our lives are reduced to visiting
doctors and clinics, keeping track of medication and therapy schedules, noting how we are feeling today and worrying about how we'll be tomorrow. When so much of our life
becomes focused on illness and its treatment, our daily routines can
seem to be quite empty and meaningless. Certainly there is little
room for joy in a lifestyle like this.

In the previous chapters, you've discovered that we begin to live
successfully with illness by letting go of our past perceptions of what
life should be and focusing on what is. But there is more to it than

that. Once we've moved beyond our previous expectations, we can begin reframing our lives. We do this by defining a new mission, one that takes us closer to the essential human needs that touch every person, whether rich or poor, young or old, ill or well—angel, sinner, Beauty, or Beast.

THE UNSUNG HEROES AND HEROINES

Many persons have a wrong idea of what constitutes true happiness. It is not attained through self-gratification but through fidelity to a worthy purpose.

Helen Keller

Finding those essential ingredients that give our lives meaning and purpose is perhaps the most deeply personal issue we will ever address, since it involves looking inward and listening to our hearts. It requires that we reaffirm our commitments to ourselves, reclaim our love for ourselves, and come to a deeper understanding of why we are more than our illnesses.

For many people, the mission that gives their lives meaning is an internal and very private one, focused on spending high-quality time with their family and closest friends. For others, it may be the pursuit of an artistic venture or even the building of a new business. And for still others it may be the quest for inner peace that comes through spiritual studies.

My own mission started in the 1980s, when I founded The MS Initiative. As I look back on it, this project was one of the most wonderful and exciting gifts I have ever received, a blessing that grew out of the challenge of my illness.

When I think of the hundreds of others I've known who looked at their lives after being diagnosed with a serious illness or physical impairment and found personal missions that made them whole, I am deeply touched. Many of us have not only overcome considerable obstacles but have found missions—sometimes in public service, sometimes in very private activities—that not only helped us cope with illness but actually led us to a way of life that was more fulfilling than what we had prior to our illness.

Over the years, I have been fascinated by the stories of people like Jim Brady, the driving force behind the controversial Brady gun control bill, who was shot in the head during the assassination attempt on President Reagan. Though he suffered brain damage that has limited his physical mobility and made it difficult for him to speak, since the shooting Jim and his wife, Sarah, have become the nation's most powerful and effective lobbyists on gun control. Through this terrible incident that came close to ending his life, Jim Brady discovered the deep satisfaction of being committed to public service at a level even more significant than before the shooting.

Life can only be understood backwards.
It must be lived forwards.

Søren Kierkegaard

We all know about celebrities like the late tennis champion Arthur Ashe, who, upon discovering that he had AIDS, founded a school to benefit young tennis hopefuls who might otherwise be unable to afford the coaching necessary to compete in world-class tennis. We know of basketball's great "Magic" Johnson, who, upon receiving a positive HIV diagnosis, started a successful outreach program to educate young people about "safe sex." But there are hundreds of thousands of ordinary people like you and me, people who are not famous athletes or celebrities, who have transformed their lives through their personal missions.

For several years before the terrible automobile accident that left him paralyzed, Joe Lohrman had a company that processed health insurance claims for large corporations. His real job was to find ways to reject or delay claims, to confuse and discourage patients so that they would either put off or drop their claims. Following the accident, and having worked extremely hard in his physical rehabilitation, but still dependent on his wheelchair, Joe had a very different perspective on the work he had been doing. He turned his attention to public service. He now offers seminars and consulting to help patients with difficult health insurance claims get the payments they deserve without delay. Of this mission of service, he says, "It's a thrill to finally use what I know to help people."

Another example that comes to mind is Ina Marx. Now in her seventies, she escaped the menace of Nazi Germany in the 1930s. But in the 1950s, trapped in a burning building, she was forced to leap from the third story. She fractured her spine and pelvis, and doctors predicted she would never walk again. In despair, she was soon addicted to prescription drugs and cigarettes, and became increasingly obese. Twice she attempted suicide. Then she discovered yoga. Through the mental, spiritual, and physical disciplines it involved, she regained her life and took on a mission to teach others with serious physical injuries how to employ yoga in their recovery. At seventy, she is slim and energetic, with a body that is as firm and flexible as that of a thirty-year-old. Now a lecturer and yoga teacher, she is also the author of a book called *Fitness for the Unfit*, which carries her message to a wide and grateful readership.

ORDINARINESS IS A PRIOR CONDITION TO GOD

Angels can fly because they take themselves lightly.

G. K. Chesterton

While these stories involving highly visible activities in the world can be an inspiration to us, it's also important to understand that the kind of mission we're going to be discussing in this chapter does not necessarily involve starting a large organization or becoming a political crusader. There are tens of thousands of other unsung heroes we never hear about, whose personal growth and deep fulfillment in the face of serious illness is no less impressive. I know of one woman whose mission is the planting and care of a lovely flower garden that brightens the lives of friends and those who pass by her front yard. I know of another woman with a serious illness who has opened her heart and established a telephone hot line to help those who have just received an unhappy diagnosis; she is able to counsel them, answer questions, and bring emotional comfort through the very trying times immediately following a medical diagnosis.

Life Skill #22

Keeping your mission to yourself is not so much secretive as it is sacred. Consider it a beautiful plant. Keep the roots (the essence of the mission) deep within yourself, and let the world share in its fruits.

It is certainly true that when we are in pain and fear, the idea of finding a mission in life may be the furthest thing from our minds, yet such a focus is profoundly healing. It can become the source of peace and personal fulfillment far beyond most people's imaginings. Through experiencing our feelings and letting go of our past perceptions of what life should be, and then having the willingness to move ahead, we discover a higher purpose in spirit. From this we are naturally uplifted, with our healing journey taking a direction toward renewed compassion for ourselves and others. It is here that illness ceases to dominate our lives.

As we've already discussed in previous chapters, to live successfully with illness we must choose life now. Don't put off your search for a mission until you "feel better." Now is the right time to begin living each moment fully, loving yourself well. This is not a fantasy or a remote possibility, for most of us, ill or well, it is a personal salvation.

WHY WE SEEK A LIFE MISSION

Although men are accused of not knowing their own weakness, yet perhaps few know their own strength. It is in men as in soils when sometimes there is a vein of gold which the owner knows not of.

Jonathan Swift

Richard Nelson Bolles's book, *How to Find Your Mission in Life*, answers the question of why we should seek a life mission. He says that when we search for a mission, we are really looking for reassurance that we are making the world a better place, and that when we leave this life, the world will be "a little poorer." We all want to feel we are making a contribution to the world, even as we improve the quality of our own lives.

It is wonderful to feel that beyond eating, sleeping, working, having a family, and growing older, we were set here on earth for a purpose. But how does one go about this search? Kahlil Gibran often said that such a journey is an "oasis of the heart," which cannot be reached only through the mind. It takes the total person to find one's mission. Above all, we need to trust the wisdom of the heart, to know that the only way to measure the value of our mission is by the degree of love and commitment we experience when we're engaged in that mission. With our hearts committed to our work, it does not matter whether we are managing the expansion of a university or tending a tiny flower garden in our own backyards; the most important aspect of the mission is that we do it as an expression of love.

It is important not to lose sight of our vitality and passionate involvement in life, regardless of what we choose to do. At our darkest moments we may ask, "Why bother? What's the point?" Or we argue, "I'm not feeling well today. I'll start on a day when I'm better." And with these words you're tempted to close the book. But I encourage you to have a little willingness, despite the disappointment, or the pain you may be feeling, or the overwhelming odds, or your failing courage or waning inner strength. If you have read this far, you can rest assured that you are already following the path that will take you closer to your mission and closer to living successfully with your illness.

IDENTIFYING YOUR MISSION

The greatest thing in this world is not so much where we are, but in what direction we are moving.

Oliver Wendell Holmes

Most of us don't discover our life mission in a few hours or even a few days, though there are certainly stories of people suddenly getting a vision of their mission through a dream or in a flash of insight. For most of us, however, a clear picture of our mission comes about only through the effort of looking very closely at our lives and following the wisdom of our hearts.

Soon after my diagnosis, the question that dominated all my waking hours, as well as my dreams, was "What am I going to do with the rest of my life now?" I felt that the proverbial rug had quite brutally been pulled out from under my feet, and I was flailing about trying to find a direction, a reason for living.

I spent a good deal of time thinking about what had had meaning for me in my past. I looked not so much at the specific activity or career role involved as the broader, underlying themes of what I had found fulfilling. I soon realized that service had always been important to me. Way back in the sixth grade, I'd gotten my first taste of this as the captain of the safety patrol. At overnight camp I was a leader of the Blue team. In 1970, I led peaceful candlelight demonstrations for the slain students at Kent State. More recently, I'd served on the task force of Philadelphia's Mayor's Commission for Women. I'd facilitated hundreds of self-awareness seminars, led corporate seminars on enhancing creativity and innovation in business, and in 1992 I thoroughly familiarized myself with the Americans with Disabilities Act, legislation sponsored by the Equal Employment Opportunity Commission.

When I began looking at these activities, I didn't at first see a common purpose. But then what began to emerge was a common intention—they were all activities that I believed, with all my heart, could make a worthwhile contribution to our world. Even more than that, however, was how each opportunity became a positive stepping stone of experience. Turning my attention to that underlying intention, it did not take me long to come up with the idea for The MS Initiative. Almost immediately, my feelings about my life changed. No longer focused on the legs that no longer supported me or the tremors that make it impossible to do my artwork or even type a letter, I knew that I could make my contribution. I could transcend physical boundaries when I looked for opportunities to serve from my heart.

As I set out to define the organization's goals, I drew upon the experiences of my own healing. I saw the organization as a way to affirm that self-support, acceptance, forgiveness, loyalty to one's own higher purpose, and unconditional loving were inherent in all healing. Within this definition of goals, illness was seen not as a stopping point but, on the contrary, as a motivator, an opportunity for expansion rather than contraction. We with multiple sclerosis became warriors, but our sword was the power of the heart. Our armor was the courageous spirit, serving selflessly, with strength and purpose. Stretching beyond our physical limitations, we rediscovered dignity in the face of fear, uncertainty, pain, and the physical, mental, and emotional constraints imposed by illness.

Simply view yourself as a pioneer, in the long journey of increasing consciousness. We started millions of years ago. No doubt we will not finish tomorrow.

Ken Keyes, Jr.

THE LIVELINESS OF YOUR MISSION

Here is the test to find whether your mission on earth is finished. If you're alive, it isn't.

Richard Bach

One of our greatest allies and resources in finding our mission is within ourselves in the form of our own inner child. In her book *Living Beyond Fear*, Jeanne Segal, Ph.D., states, "Our [inner] child is our partner in becoming wholly alive as we exchange a few gray areas of non-feeling for a full palette of emotions. Our process of healing naturally leads us to express all human emotions—from rage to ecstasy—as part of our daily living." In a very real way, it is this full palette of emotions that we bring to the mission, drawing on the strengths and aliveness of the inner child as our partner.

It is my belief that our mission often becomes a container for all that we are feeling. For me, the mission of The MS Initiative, as well as this book, was a container for the rage that was triggered for me by the cold neurologist who told me, "Too bad you're so cute. You'll be in a wheelchair, you know!" It was a container for the forgiveness, unconditional love, self-affirmation, and devotion that came later, and which continue to awaken and expand.

When our mission contains and expresses all of these seemingly divergent components, we can transform our rage into positive action, from the emptiness of guilt, blame, bitterness, disappointment, and pain toward correcting or healing something that isn't right. From the vantage point of our chosen mission, we can observe situations that need attention and turn energy toward changing them for the better. We can take action, doing something to heal or soothe ourselves and others.

A Mission from the Heart

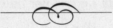

The question is not whether we will die,
but how we will live.

Joan Borysenko

I am often asked, "Is it enough that my mission is spending quality time with my family?" Yes, of course. Once again, it is not the magnitude or number of people you affect that counts in your mission. What's important is the engagement of the heart. The mission of one man I know is doing jigsaw puzzles with his grandchildren. Paralyzed following a stroke, he and three of his grandchildren get together at least twice a week to do puzzles together; but the real mission becomes obvious only when you see them together. Beyond the puzzles, there is a communion of hearts that literally lights up the room.

I met a woman in California who has Parkinson's disease. She continues her work as a psychotherapist, thanks to having her office in her home. In her spare time she has planted one of the most beautiful flower gardens I have ever seen. Living in California, she has included many exotic plants, such as orchids and bird-of-paradise. Her garden has become a place of healing not only for her but for her clients, and even strangers who pause at her fence to enjoy her artistry.

In his book *How to Find Your Mission in Life*, Richard Nelson Bolles suggests that searching for a mission "inevitably leads us to God." As you begin to fully appreciate the experience of having a mission, you may very well begin to recognize that perhaps there is a Higher Power than our own selves that participates in this process. When we ask to be of service, we may find someone such as a retired parent, an infirm cousin, or a homeless stranger seeking shelter. Maybe that is how you serve, and you may even begin to experience God as your co-creator. When we direct our particular skills and personal gifts toward a specific activity that touches others—even just one person—in a way that makes their lives a little better, we have found our mission. And in this process of asking to be of service, we have acknowledged God's presence in our lives.

INTENTION AND MISSION

Man's mind, once stretched by a new idea, never regains its original dimensions.

Oliver Wendell Holmes

As you set out to identify your mission, it can be helpful to make a distinction between intention and method. For example, while your intention might be to get to the airport, there might be many methods for getting there; you might go by cab, bus, or train, for example. In the same way, there are many methods for reaching the intention of one's life mission. Let me explain.

When I first became ill, I began looking at all the different activities that had brought real pleasure into my life. I thought of how much I'd enjoyed being a crossing guard in the sixth grade, being on the Blue team at camp, organizing candlelight vigils at Kent State, designing and art directing the activities for Philadelphia's three hundredth birthday celebration, facilitating corporate seminars, and being on various public service committees. Each of these, I soon saw, was a different method for achieving the same intention. The intention that ran through all these activities had to do with service—that is, being of service to others. I then asked, in what way can I continue to enjoy and express this intention now that I have MS? And the answer came very quickly: through another form of service. First I found my mission in The MS Initiative. Later, that work carried me further, to write this book, knowing that it, too, would minister and be of service to others.

Our mission is always found not by looking at our methods but by getting to know our intentions. Arthur Ashe found his intention through inspiring others, stimulating their imaginations to reach for the edge of human capabilities. Every time he competed in a tournament, this intention drove him to reach into himself and attain the highest levels of human potential. Then, when his illness forced him to stop playing, he founded a school where, in another way, the same intention could be expressed—this time in providing up-and-coming athletes an opportunity to be coached by people who would help them attain the very best in themselves.

To identify your own mission, first think back to moments in your childhood, as well as later in your life, when you were involved in an activity where you felt excited, alive, and fully engaged. Look for times when your will and your heart were working in harmony toward achieving a single goal or activity. In his groundbreaking work on optimal human performance, the psychologist Abraham Maslow called such moments "peak experiences." To have a peak experience, you don't need to be a champion athlete or a high-visibility celebrity. Not by any means! Maslow said that we all have these peak experiences, whether it's in a world-class competition, listening to music in our own living rooms, baking a birthday cake for a family member, or walking on the beach during a beautiful sunset. Again, the fullness of our heart is our only measure of such experiences. Look to it. It is your strength.

In his landmark book, *Toward a Psychology of Being*, Maslow wrote that when one is having a peak experience, "the powers of the person come together in a particularly efficient and intensely enjoyable way . . . [and we are] . . . more integrated and less split, more open for experience." As you look for the peak experiences in your life, call upon the aid of your inner child. He or she is that part of you that knows how it feels to have a peak experience. Your inner child is always engaged in these experiences, open and vitally alive, giving and receiving fully, even when the mission seems, on the surface, to be quite "grown up."

I am reminded of a time at overnight camp when my friend Joyce and I spontaneously jumped off a loft in a huge barn filled with grain. I was nine or ten. I jumped repeatedly and enthusiastically, jumping over and over and over again until I was exhausted and laughing hysterically. I still remember how the counselors were flailing their arms, screaming and shouting for me to stop!

There is something in this experience that reminds me of my mission today: unwavering determination, persistence, risk taking, freedom of expression, enthusiasm, and passion for life.

Once you have recalled three or four activities of this kind, look for the intention they share. Be careful that you don't get sidetracked by the methods you employed for achieving that intention. For example, I once loved to run on the beach. Today, of course, I can't do that. But running on the beach was only the method. Beyond this was the intention, and in this case my intention had to do with a particular kind of relationship I experienced with nature. That intention is still mine to enjoy, anytime I want it. Anytime I wish, I can bask in the presence of God, and see His hand in all His works, be it a fiery sunset or the joy of completing another chapter of my book. Nature is all around us. We are not just observers of it but full participants. Our joy in this can never be taken from us.

Now, taking your full life into account, with love, acceptance, and forgiveness, as we have described in the previous pages, look at the ways you can shape your key intentions into a new mission. My friend Hal recently told me about a woman in one of his workshops who had been a dancer, but the disease lupus had caused a deterioration in the cartilage of her hips, making it difficult for her to even walk. This woman, now Sister Loretta, was very spiritual and had joined a contemplative order of nuns of the Catholic church. But for years she had mourned the loss of her legs and had deeply missed the experience of dancing. There had even been times when she had been so angry and frustrated by her illness, and what she felt it had taken from her, that she raged at God, proclaiming that it wasn't fair.

I hear and behold God in every object,
yet I understand God not in the least.

Walt Whitman

In the workshop, and in work she did on her own following it, she got in touch with her intention. In all her dance experiences, there had been the feeling of celebrating God. In a dream one night, it suddenly came to her that she had always celebrated God in all her work. When she woke up that morning, she also remembered that as a child she used to write poems and small vignettes that did the same thing; in fact, these poems and vignettes were themselves like dances. In the word play of these pieces, there was rhythm and motion. There was music in her phrasing that sailed and pirouetted. That afternoon, she recited some of her old poems to her friends. Once again she was a dancer, not with her legs this time but with the goodness of her heart, expressed through her words.

Life Skill #23

When we give to someone, something, or some cause greater than ourselves, we feel transcendent and expanded. The person, thing, or cause we give to becomes greater for our gift, and—seemingly violating the law of physics—we become greater too.

This story seems to me to offer such an inspiring example of how the human spirit finds expression and deep satisfaction not just in one form or method but in an infinite variety of ways. It is also a reminder that the truth of our intention is always found in the essence of our love, kindness, laughter, wisdom—in a smile or moment of sharing our own delight with others.

One of the most important reasons for being alive is the child within us all.

Bruce Davis, Ph.D.

NURTURING YOURSELF THROUGH YOUR MISSION

There are only two things you must do in this lifetime: Be of service to others as much as possible, and polish your inner being to its fullest radiance.

Masami Saionji

When we look carefully at people with clear missions in their lives, we find that while they feel that what they are doing gives their life meaning and purpose, they are also deeply nurtured in return. The nurturing comes not by asking service from others—though it might come naturally through the mission in any case—but as an integral part of the activity of serving. It is useful, therefore, to take a look at what nurtures you and make certain that it is in some way satisfied through your mission.

Usually, what truly nurtures us are the simple pleasures of life, experiences we might take for granted if we didn't actually take time to stop and think about them. For this reason, I suggest that you take some time to just relax and in a heartfelt way ask yourself to think about the moments in your life when you feel truly nurtured. Then list these moments in your journal. Take time with this. Don't rush it. Too often we have such a fast pace in life that we completely forget those fleeting moments that are so rich and fulfilling. Here's a list of my own nurturing pleasures, most of which satisfy my mission of being at one with nature:

- The beach house at Barnegat Light on a cool day in September
- The smell of a fire in my fireplace
- God as my partner
- Lazy Sunday mornings with Michael by my side
- Listening to the saxophone and jazz by Grover Washington, Jr.
- Silk lingerie
- Touching my friend Elizabeth's cheek
- Autumn leaves in vivid colors
- The sound of wind chimes

- My cats, Lucy and Sasha
- A Libra moon
- White roses sent to me for no special reason
- Crystals catching the sunlight
- A warm rainy day in October
- An amethyst sunset in the Badlands
- Sid—my teddy bear
- Speaking with my precious inner child
- An affectionate hug from my friend John

Focus on the quality of feelings that you associate with these nurturing pleasures. In what ways are the same, or similar, feelings experienced in your mission? I find, for example, that when I am writing, many of the same nurturing experiences come into play. For instance, there are many moments when I strongly feel God as my partner, and when I do, my energy feels balanced and focused. Often, too, my cat Lucy leaps up on my computer monitor, her tail draping down across the screen. Though her swishing tail can become a distraction, to say the least, there is something nurturing in her presence so I cannot bring myself to shoo her away.

If you do not discover that some of the simple pleasures are already incorporated into your mission, I would be very surprised. But if they're not, look for ways to bring them in. Adjust your mission so that you are nurtured and gently filled.

Close your eyes and you will see clearly.
Cease to listen and you will hear truth.
Be silent and your heart will sing.
Seek no contact and you will find union.
Be still and you will move on the tide of the Spirit.
Be gentle and you will need no strength.
Be patient and you will achieve all things.
Be humble and you will remain entire.

Ancient Chinese poem

SELF-APPRECIATION AND MISSION

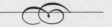

Throughout this book we have explored self-appreciation and the importance of loving ourselves well. Unless we truly understand and live with appreciation for ourselves, we cannot give wholly with love to the world. Very often, in fact, it is our lack of self-appreciation that robs us of the experience of feeling that our lives have purpose. Our missions bring into sharp focus not only our special gifts but our own recognition of those gifts. In the process, we embrace ourselves, our spirit, the love that is extended through us by God—and in this embrace is the most powerful form of healing in the world.

Bernie Siegel, M.D., has often said, "Without self-love it is hard to fight for one's life!" I would take that even a step further: without self-love there can be no sense of purpose, no way to give and receive, no way to experience ourselves as nurturing and being nurtured. We are robbed of the mission through which our lives become complete.

As we close this chapter, bring your self-appreciation into focus. Think of the ways you bring your inner strength, clarity, enthusiasm, inspiration, willingness, acceptance, and gratitude to your mission. Take a moment to acknowledge to yourself the positive difference you make in other people's lives, particularly as it is expressed in your mission. Give thanks to the inner child who is the source of your varied palette of color, the rhythmic dance that fuels your inner spirit. Appreciate the shining light that is your mission, illuminating your path and providing a beacon that, in some small but important way, helps others find their way.

The purpose is not to heal, only to love.
It is the love that heals.

Gurudev (Yogi Amrit Desai)

Part Three

LIVING IN

GRACE

Life is a song—sing it.

Life is a game—play it.

Life is a challenge—meet it.

Life is a dream—realize it.

Life is a sacrifice—offer it.

Life is love—enjoy it.

Sai Baba

7

The Inner Path
of Mastership

You are a child of the universe,
No less than the trees and the stars;
You have a right to be here.
And whether or not it is clear to you,
No doubt the universe
Is unfolding as it should.

Max Ehrmann

To suffer is not enough. Through the experiences of illness we can shift our perspective of what is important and what is not. We can learn to touch the wonders of life beyond the suffering. There is a part of us—dare we call it the soul?—that allows us to identify with life beyond the suffering, to dissociate from the discomfort and limitation of the physical body. And when we can pay attention and open ourselves to receive, we discover that the wonders of life are all around us, everywhere, all the time. We are held, if only for brief moments, in the gentler, drifting processes that are the qualities of the soul. We bask in God's gift of our breath, of colors, textures, sounds. We hear the deeper, fuller, more loving and profound music of the spheres; we feel the breathtaking joy of an amethyst sunset; we see the soul in the eyes of a laughing baby. John-Roger says that devotion may express itself as "Lord, here I am to help, to be helped, to share and be one with all." I take this to mean "I don't have to be all things to all people. I'm not even going to try. I'm just going to be me."

Through illness I have come to see that God's ways are always simple, direct, free of pretense and illusion. I have come to know that the essence of who I am is far more than my body. I have a clear sense of the illusions and negative projections of my body, but regardless of how I am feeling or of how others might perceive me, I know that within this body is God's creation, which is a beautiful, lovable, and loving being.

I have learned to see the human body as the vehicle to anchor our awareness and growth, and when we create unconditional acceptance for our body, regardless of illness, consciousness is freed to explore realities beyond the physical world. And then we can truly say that those who are able to make this journey beyond illness, and beyond the physical form, are truly the chosen ones. In this respect, my illness has been my greatest teacher, causing me to reflect, in quiet moments, on the very real possibility that it has been a gift rather than a misfortune.

Through observation, I have developed the ability to distance myself when things got rough, to focus on the positive and shut out everything else. Seeking the higher truth became a survival technique for me, a way to find value and goodness in whatever situation I was going through. Regardless of the circumstances, the skills of observation helped me clarify my mission and find meaning beyond the suffering.

For as long as I can remember, even far back into my childhood, my imagination has allowed me to take wing, allowing me to express myself creatively. I was not only able to fantasize but to bring many of my fantasies into reality.

Amazing grace, how sweet the sound
that saved a soul like me.
I once was lost, but now I'm found,
was blind, but now I see.

American spiritual

In her book *Guilt Is the Teacher, Love Is the Lesson*, Joan Borysenko, Ph.D., defines Grace as "a living act and expression of the natural laws by which love extends itself. The impetus to make the hero's journey, to search for the Self, to be reconciled with God, is an act of Grace. Grace comes unearned as a free, unsought gift." As in the old spiritual, Grace restores our spiritual vision so that we can see where we're going. I believe that illness can provide us with the foundation for discovering Grace and for awakening to the reality beyond the indulgence with our physical existence.

Not long ago, trend watcher Tom Wolfe predicted that "moral fever" would rule the nineties, that we would embark on a desperate search for values. In a 1994 *Newsweek* poll, 76 percent of adults agreed that the United States is in moral and spiritual decline, and the craving for "virtue" is creating a new class of leaders in a national obsession. "The New Frontier of the 90's is an inner one. Character building is mostly a matter of private quests and private struggles," declares the author Peggy Noonan, reflecting the theme of her book *Life, Liberty and the Pursuit of Happiness*. "We have to help each other out of this hole. This is a country full of prayer groups—and that's what they are for."

Americans are agreeing that there are universally accepted principles of good character—"virtues"—and society is failing to teach them anymore, says *Newsweek* magazine in a June 13, 1994 article "The Politics of Virtues." It now seems painfully clear to most Americans that none of the traditional institutions is doing the job.

Clearly, we are experiencing a rebirth of early sixties optimism, a belief that we can nurture an American dream of one day having an emotionally harmonious, all-inclusive sense of "us"—a way of life based on peace and love instead of fear, guilt, unworthiness, hurt feelings, and discouragement. In an April 8, 1991 article "The Simple Life," *Time* magazine referred to this revolution in progress as "Americans returning to basics and simpler pleasures, redis-covering the joys of home life, basic values, spirituality, and things that last."

As people learning to live successfully with illness, we are at the center of this movement, *pioneers* focused once again on embracing basic principles, values, and spirituality. No one knows better than us the importance of focusing our lives in these ways, through accep-tance, loving, compassion, and forgiveness. In all that we confront in physical suffering and limitation, we discover the path to values that are both eternal and comforting.

- As we free the frightened and innocent child within, we begin to reclaim the inner peace that is our birthright.

- As we free ourselves from the concept that our identity is limited to our personalities—what we think, say, do, or how we feel today—we feel ourselves living more fully through that part of us known as the soul.

- As we accept and honor ourselves as we are right now, we discover that our true freedom is found in the spirit, not in our bodies, emotions, or minds.

- As we accept our own lives, rather than judging them for what they are not, we also accept others for who they are instead of who we might want them to be.

- As we learn to receive God's love for us, we discover that we are all joined in our hearts as One.

- As we begin to see that all of life is our teacher, we see every event as a mirror, providing us with a clear image of the next step in our path of personal growth.

- Through the practice of forgiveness we discover that love is the most powerful healer.

- In recognizing that our true identity is spiritual, we discover that we can depend on and trust the Spirit to guide us, provid-ing unlimited wisdom, clarity, and love, far beyond anything the personality itself could ever provide.

- In the acceptance of the negative aspects of ourselves, the parts that we would rather reject or pretend don't exist, we discover our humanness and bring light and peace both to our inner

LIVING IN GRACE / 203

selves and to the global community of which we are an integral part.

The path of Grace begins when we choose to affirm our love for ourselves by pursuing a simpler life, one with deeper meaning, rather than reacting to our physical or emotional circumstances with anger, fear, doubt, guilt, or depression. When we are in pain or have just received news that frightens us, it can seem that we have no choice, that anger, fear, and doubt are natural and automatic reactions. But through the practices we've been exploring in these pages, we gain the power of choice—even in the face of our greatest challenges. That power is the source of our inner authority and strength; it is the expression of Grace in our lives.

Does this mean that we cease to experience those feelings we might judge as "negative," or that we are always in control of our emotions? No, there is not a day that I don't fall down emotionally. However, the better I get to know myself and how I relate to the qualities of character we've been exploring here, the faster I am able to pick myself up again—often doing so immediately. Grace is always extended, something that becomes clearer each time I remind myself that healing is an ongoing process, never a final destination. In recognizing this I let go. Through Grace I can accept that healing, like the opening of a flower, is a gradual awakening that we cannot rush.

As we learn to reach out for the Grace that is always extended, we begin asking new questions. Instead of seeing ourselves as the victims of adversity, we ask ourselves what lessons are being extended to us in this new challenge. We begin to look at ourselves as being on the hero's journey, in search this time not of the Golden Fleece but of our Self and our relationship to God or that Higher Power of our belief. As we work the processes described in this book, we learn that the way out of adversity—be it an illness or other personal challenge—often begins with surrendering to it. We learn that acceptance and surrender are the only way through; the sense of surrender I feel at such times is very much like looking out my window and seeing the flowers budding and knowing that I need do nothing. It is in God's hands. This, too, is Grace.

In truth, we always walk the path of Grace. If we don't see that path or the lights that life puts out to guide us along the way, it is only because we have closed our own eyes to it or have clouded our minds and emotions so that we cannot experience it. As I accept and forgive, as I drop self-criticism and harshness, regardless of pain, spasticity, discomfort, and feelings of unworthiness, I once again awaken, opening my eyes to the path that Grace offers me.

Our idea of God tells us more about ourselves than about Him.

Thomas Merton

Too often we mistakenly think that we can gain peace by controlling the physical world and all it represents—our sensations, our thoughts, our judgments, our emotions, our bodies. There can be little argument that this is not entirely untrue—for without some exercise of control we might wander into the path of a speeding truck and be struck down. But beyond the prison bars of the body, emotions, and mind *we discover the freedom of consciousness that is pure soul.*

As we continue to pursue our journey of lifelong learning, we discover how to share our inner light. Since we are mirrors to one another, we find that same light reflected in others as they discover it reflected in us. Life becomes joyful, and the disturbances we associate with our physical beings gradually become less compelling, less the center of our lives.

There is no direct way to get love. It comes from giving and expecting nothing in return. When love comes from giving, it comes to you as Grace.

Gurudev (Yogi Amrit Desai)

MIRRORS OF SELF-APPRECIATION

As we walk in Grace, we recognize the best in ourselves mirrored back to us through the best in others. Just as we attract light into our lives as we recognize the light in others and appreciate them, so it is important to do the same for ourselves. To do this, think about the people you most admire, people who inspire you and give you strength. As you think about them or enjoy their presence, recognize that they are a mirror, reflecting back the same positive aspects in yourself. What you see in them is being reflected back to you from your own inner being. Acknowledge this important truth and appreciate yourself for your positive impact in this relationship.

Grace is found in taking the time to express love, respect, and nourishment for ourselves and learning to receive this form of self-appreciation. If we have been judgmental and critical of ourselves in the past—and who has not been?—it may take some time for us to get used to this kind of feedback. It can be helpful to actually make a list, from time to time, of the positive qualities we recognize in ourselves and refer to these when giving this self-appreciation. It seems that most of us neglect ourselves when we are expressing appreciation. My friend Hal Bennett refers to this kind of conscious self-appreciation as "polishing the mirror so that we can better see our own best qualities reflected back to us."

No joy can equal the joy of serving others.

Sai Baba

The Grace we are seeking is found in a state of wellness that is far more than a reversal of disease or injury. The wellness we seek is a process of reconnecting with ourselves—a process of learning to listen and trust those inner resources that lead us to the peace of mind we all seek. It is found in learning to hear the highest truths as they are reflected back to us in conversations with others, or perhaps in the lyrics of a song, or in the question of a small child, or in an unexpected letter from a dear friend. It is the answer we find through our inner stillness, when we access a source of wisdom beyond the limits of our physical being.

FAITHING—GRACE IN ACTION

Faithing works here and now. It acknowledges that there's a plan at work, and that the plan is being perfectly executed. We may not like it, but it's being perfectly executed just the same. Faithing is flowing with what's going on, whatever that may be.

John-Roger

Faith is an important part of living in Grace with our illness. But faith, like love, is an active, ongoing process that is best understood as a verb, a word that describes an action. In the bestselling book, *Do-It!*, John-Roger continues to say that "faithing is trusting that everything will work out for the highest good of all." When we have an illness, there are few beliefs more challenging than this one. After all, being ill is hardly the way we would want things to be. But with faith, we realize that our opinions, wants, and desires, our beliefs about the way things ought to be are not necessarily what will work out for the best in the bigger picture. One of the great lessons we must learn is that what we perceive as disorder may be only a small portion of a bigger order we simply do not have the capacity to see. Faithing is trusting in this higher order, putting aside our personal agendas, our shoulds, musts, opinions, and beliefs, and moving into the flow of what is actually happening right now. With faithing we let go of our own limited judgments and put our lives in Spirit's hands.

In *You Can't Afford the Luxury of a Negative Thought*, John-Roger says, "We may not like the way things are turning out but with faith we realize that our opinion and desire about how we think it should be aren't necessarily the way it will work out best."

Having put our lives in Spirit's hands, we can begin to see their richness more clearly. We notice the splendor of the trees in autumn, the spectacle of the world's new birth in the spring. We look into the face of a close friend or loved one and see our Self mirrored in them. During these special holy moments we enter a state of Grace that is always available to us.

LIVING IN GOD'S HOLY THOUGHTS (LIGHT)

We attend in silence and joy. This is the day when healing comes to us. This is the day when separation ends, and we remember who we really are.

A Course in Miracles

When I am too busy thinking about picking up the dry cleaning, remembering cat litter, the balance in my checking account, doctors' appointments, spring planting, or how my physical therapy is going; when I am enjoying managing my home, my long-term mission in life; or how I am nurturing my support relationships, it is a challenge to stay present while enjoying a wonderful meal or making love to my husband. When my mind is wandering, or flitting like a nervous bird from one thing to the next, there is little room for Grace.

There are times when I must yank on my reins, stop, and force myself to be reminded of my blessings. At such times, I look out my office window at the budding trees and early spring foliage. I must force myself to slow down and enjoy a most glorious sunset. I remind myself to be silent and dwell only in the present moment, knowing it is the only moment there is. In the moment we find our blessings. And with our blessings come our gratitude and contentment, which also exist in the present, with the self-love that naturally accompanies them.

Martin Luther King, Jr., once said, "Faith is the opening of all sides and every level of one's life to the divine inflow." Our blessings are found in realizing that God's perfect plan is revealed to us in all things. We move forward with Grace in accepting our goodness, determination, and willingness to live our lives moment by moment as a demonstration of our love.

The role of faith in our lives is very clearly described in the Bible. Jesus said, for example, that if we have the faith of a mustard seed we can move mountains. The analogy being drawn here is that from a single mustard seed can grow acres and acres of beautiful yellow mustard, a veritable sea of color that moves over the earth. In the same way, our single seed of faith may spread throughout our own lives.

We move into Grace when we are no longer attached to the outcome of healing our bodies; we are, however, inspired by the realization that our healing has more to do with awakening to the process of self-acceptance and forgiveness, bathing in the inner peace of our spiritual growth. We move into Grace when we discover the power of transformation that every illness offers us.

THE BLESSING

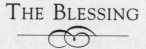

Each day I find I must remind myself to let go of that which is not me, forgiving myself for self-judgments and allowing that which is truly me to unfold. In my journal there is an entry that I have flagged with a bookmark so that I can find it quickly when I feel stuck. It is a reminder to me that I can move on from self-judgment. It says:

Michael is home sick with the flu today and I'm doing my best to make chicken soup. I can barely walk without painfully leaning on counters, walls, the refrigerator, my kitchen table —anything for support. Something inside me begins to break. I sob and sob, "I can't even make you chicken soup! I'm such a bad wife!" I cry as he sweetly holds me, rocking. I am being unfair and cruel to myself, he reminds me, confusing who I am with my judgments of self-worth, my inability to make chicken soup, the degenerating discs in my lower spine, and my habitual negative thinking. I am confusing the state of my body and its symptoms with my identity. I am reminded, instead, that who

I am is unconditional love and forgiveness, to do what I can, moment to moment, day by day, step by step, to make this world a better place, following the guidance of God's spirit within me and around me.

Reading this, once again, I forgive myself my judgmental thoughts, feelings, and behaviors, reminded of how important it is to recognize my humanness in all this. I am blessed with my husband, Michael, whose love and genuine support help me affirm my conviction that neither my physical body nor the things I say, do, or feel are true reflections of my self-worth. Beyond my negative thoughts and feelings, there are a great many blessings to which I daily give thanks through gratitude.

THE ATTITUDE OF GRATITUDE

Shall we make a new rule of life tonight: always try to be a little kinder than is necessary.

Sir James M. Barrie

Through our inner and outer expression of gratitude, we thank God for even the simplest of pleasures—the haunting song of the mourning dove, the sound of a gentle rain on the roof, the brilliant colors of a spring day, the intimate support of friends and loved ones, the first twinkling star of the evening—even the discomfort associated with our bodies. Gratitude reminds us to find our happiness in exceptional things, mundane things, the good things, the so-so things—even the terrible things.

You cannot prevent the birds of sorrow from flying over your head, but you can prevent them from building nests in your hair.

Chinese proverb

In quiet moments, I recognize that I have a choice; I can look with gratitude upon the information about my life that comes to me in the form of muscle spasms, headache, lower back pain, tremors, disappointment, anger, grief, fear, confusion, doubt, and self-judgment. In all of these I find lessons to wake myself up, reduce stress, live more fully in the moment, rest, forgive, and be true to my intentions to love myself, love God, and serve others. Each ache and pain, each moment of doubt or fear is part of an automatic feedback system, directing me to pay attention, to appreciate all that is so magnificent in my life that I may tend to forget or take for granted.

I know that when I take the time to be grateful, I naturally become more loving, forgiving, and respectful toward the wonder of the human body and the recognition of the spark of the Divine Spirit that is in all of us. In gratitude, I find that I can more easily look for only the good in all people and all events, and leave the responsibility of fixing the broken pieces to God. It is then that I truly cease to judge my own life. And it is then that I can better see that my negative thinking, my sense of unworthiness, the pain or hurt feelings I experience are my teachers. I am then reminded of the words of a great teacher, Tarthang Tulku, who said, "Complete health and awakening are really the same."

THE WILLINGNESS TO CHANGE— ONCE AGAIN

MARY RICHARDS: It's a lousy business we're in, Mr. Grant; I quit. I'm going to Africa to work with Schweitzer.
LOU GRANT: Mary, Albert Schweitzer is dead.
MARY RICHARDS: You see what I mean, Mr. Grant? It's a lousy, lousy world.

The Mary Tyler Moore Show

Because everything in the world is our mirror, the image in the mirror changes as we change. As we develop new habits of supporting, trusting, co-creating, and loving ourselves, we will gradually begin to release and heal our own limitations. I am always amazed and delighted at how others respond when I am feeling inner peace and acceptance and love; nearly every contact with others further confirms the feelings I am experiencing. People around me seem to open up to their own power, vulnerabilities, opportunities, dreams, and commitments. So often I find that the more light I shine from within, the brighter the world seems to become all around me. I become a peacemaker in my heart and carry that peace into the world.

If the world truly is our mirror, as I believe it is, then every event occurring within it—be it territorial and religious crisis in the Middle East, starvation by hunger in Bosnia-Hercegovina and Sarajevo, racial and spousal violence in American cities, environmental pollutants, the AIDS epidemic, the grisly nightmare of Rwanda, inhumane animal testing, graffiti, the nuclear crisis in North Korea, global warming, or brutal assassinations of political leaders all over the world—all these in some way reflect a conflict raging within each of us individually and all of us collectively. Without blame, shame, grief, fear, terror, or guilt, we discover a deep willingness to change our own lives and so help to transform the world. We must never forget that in consciousness, in Spirit, we are all related, and what we heal in ourselves we automatically heal in others. We are all one.

When one has once fully entered the realm of love, the world—no matter how imperfect—becomes rich and beautiful, for it consists solely of opportunities for love.

Søren Kierkegaard

BEYOND THIS BOOK

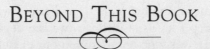

The sanctuary of the heart is the location of peace. You move into the spiritual heart to discover peace. God

speaks to you through your heart. God brings peace to
your life. You can know happiness, and you can know
love. There is nothing else worth knowing. Love is the
only channel for clear communication. And peace is the
parent of love.

John-Roger

I like to believe that the search for the inner peace that I seek in my relationship to my illness has a significance beyond my individual life. Somehow I know that in each step of the healing process we are all moving toward a way of peace that extends far beyond the short span of our own years. Not long ago I learned about the Peace Pole Project, which teaches, "War begins with thoughts of war. Peace begins with thoughts of peace." We know that peace is far more than the cessation of war. It is a thought, a dream, a commitment that we hold in our own minds.

From 1976 to 1991, the organization has been responsible for the planting of over 35,000 Peace Poles around the world, in front of schools, in parks, at churches and synagogues, at city halls and private homes. Each pole is a reminder that in seeking peace within ourselves we are making one more step to global peace. Each pole is a reminder to hold these thoughts of peace within our own minds.

On March 10, 1991, Michael and I, with the help of friends, neighbors, and loved ones, planted a four-sided Peace Pole outside our home, with a simple ceremony dedicating our individual and collective efforts to global peace. We all came away wondering what each of us could do in our private lives to contribute to peace. "First keep the peace within yourself," Thomas A. Kempis once said, "then you can also bring peace to others."

For those of us who have serious illnesses, it can be tremendously helpful to see our own search for inner peace and healing in this larger, global context. The challenge for each of us, as our world moves toward the new millennium, is to discover what is authentic, what are the deeper levels of intimacy we can develop in our relationships to ourselves, one another, and our planet. If it serves no other purpose, our learning to live successfully with illness serves in these ways. In our personal challenge, we can, in healing ourselves spiritually, give new life to the universal values of compassion, humor, love, freedom, and creative self-expression. In seeking our own peace and comfort, we join in an expression of our oneness, a psychospiritual response that transcends all our individual concerns. If illness teaches us nothing else, it is that peace, our ultimate healing, is found by going within, to the higher source of our being, cultivating our own inner peace by stopping the fighting and battles within our personal consciousness. This process is by no means a static journey. It is a journey and a mission that lasts as long as our lives.

It is the consistent choice of the path with heart which makes the warrior different from the average man. He knows that path has heart when he is one with it, when he experiences a great peace and pleasure traversing its length.

Carlos Castañeda

LIVING AS LONG AS THE MISSION REQUIRES

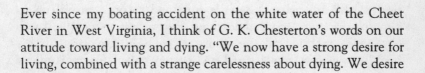

Ever since my boating accident on the white water of the Cheet River in West Virginia, I think of G. K. Chesterton's words on our attitude toward living and dying. "We now have a strong desire for living, combined with a strange carelessness about dying. We desire life like water and yet are ready to drink death like wine."

I believe that we are delivered from the fear of how much longer we have to live when we settle it in our heart that we are here until God decides we have accomplished our mission or until God decides we have a greater mission in another realm. We are here to do what we came here to do. We need not worry about anything else.

THE ZEN OF ILLNESS

We really don't have the expression of outer loving until our inner loving is there. We aren't going to have outer peace in the world until we stop having the wars inside ourselves. That's our job—to start having peace inside.

John-Roger

My friends sometimes tease me that I approach my illness in much the same way that a Zen monk approaches the everyday tasks of life, such as the proverbial routines of chopping wood and carrying water. While I certainly do not live in a monastery, there is a part of me that would have to agree there is more than a little truth in what they say. Though I might approach my illness in this way, I live and work very much in the modern world. And it is my belief that in our search for quality of life—that is, lives where we feel at peace, where our lives have meaning and purpose—we are all seeking a path that has these same goals.

I believe that my illness has taught me much that I might not have otherwise learned—at least not as quickly as I have. But I also know that I have always pursued the kinds of self-knowledge, ethics, and values that I have discovered in my present way of life.

I find that in every way I am constantly being offered opportunities to both test what I have learned and to open myself up to new self-discovery and new learning. Recently, for example, I was challenged to bring all the values we've been exploring in this book into play. Michael and I had gotten tickets for an Andreas Vollenweider concert. As was my habit, I called the concert hall several days ahead to find out about handicapped facilities, and was told there would be no problem. However, when we arrived the night of the concert we found that there was no handicapped seating or parking. I was appalled and discouraged by the facilities—or, rather, lack of them. The ladies room was down a long flight of steps, impossible for me to negotiate.

This was an opportunity to pull out every spiritual tool I'd ever learned. The Seven Personal Keys to freedom and personal peace—

Honesty, Compassion, Acceptance, Patience, Cooperation, Observation, and Loyalty—all leapt to mind. By using these actively and aggressively I was able to pull myself out of my sense of contraction and defeat and move ahead in a creative way. We got into the theater, arranged seating, and the concert began.

During intermission I needed to use the toilet. With more than a little hassle, Michael and I located a bathroom in a bar adjacent to the theater. To get there we had to thread our way through a nearly impossible obstacle course. With my trusty scooter, I wheeled briskly through a crowd of five hundred people, out the back door of the theater, down a loading ramp, out the back alley, and into the bar. Then, with a juke box pounding in my ears, smoke being blown into my face, and an entire roomful of staring eyes, Michael lifted me up, and just in time I maneuvered into a very small space—all this just to go to the bathroom! I had to bring into play all the Seven Keys, and then some. But through the keys I stood up within myself and supported myself in a way that allowed me to feel whole and strong.

In addition to the struggles with the facilities, I was confronted with a number of personal challenges that night. I bumped into a good friend from college whom I had not seen for fifteen years. This was the first time she had seen me in a wheelchair and she was shocked, necessitating an honest personal exchange that was difficult for both of us. I also ran into an old friend from a women's group to which I'd belonged twenty years before, and the editor of a magazine who'd not seen me for some time. Each of these encounters required me to consciously and deliberately make use of the Seven Personal Keys.

By using the Seven Keys, I successfully continue to live with my illness and in the process to learn from it. It isn't always easy, of course, and each time I encounter a new challenge I must remind myself that I always have a choice. I can retreat and hide from life. Or I can accept my present situation as an opportunity for further healing and growth. I surrender to the way it is and look for ways to be loving, peaceful, and receptive, knowing that out of this opportunity there invariably comes a creative solution.

As challenging as that evening was, I came away from the concert feeling that there was room in the world to be me, scooter and all, impossible facilities and all, seedy bar and all. It certainly was not the external world that made the eventual difference but the inner skills and abilities I had been given through the years and was now able to draw upon.

I believe that regardless of illness or health, we are all seeking a solid foundation upon which to build our lives. Whether we are aware of it or not, we are always looking, always learning, hopefully building our lives on values and skills that can make our own lives, and the lives of those around us, a little better, a little more peaceful, a little more prayerful. It is to those ends that I would pray this book might be of service.

I chose to end these pages with a quote from Guillaume Appollinaire:

"Come to the edge," he said.

They said, "We are afraid."

"Come to the edge," he said.

They came.

He pushed them . . .

And they flew.

For Further Reading

I am grateful to the authors of the following books for their wisdom, teachings, and the wealth of their contributions. Thank you.

HEALTH AND HEALING

Achterberg, Jeanne. *Imagery in Healing*. Boston: New Science Library, 1985.

Benson, Herbert, and Miriam Z. Klipper. *The Relaxation Response*. New York: Avon Books, 1976.

Carlson, Richard, Ph.D., and Benjamin Shield, eds. *Healers on Healing*. Los Angeles: Jeremy P. Tarcher, 1989.

Chopra, Deepak, M.D. *Perfect Health*. New York: Harmony Books, 1990.

——. *Quantum Healing*. New York: Bantam Books, 1989.

——. *Unconditional Life: Discovering the Power to Fulfill Your Dreams*. New York: Bantam Books, 1991.

Epstein, Gerald. *Healing Visualizations: Creating Health Through Imagery*. New York: Bantam Books, 1989.

Harrison, John W., M.D. *Love Your Disease*. London: Angus and Robertson, 1984.

Hay, Louise L. *You Can Heal Your Life*. Santa Monica: The Hay House, 1984.

Hutchinson, Marcia Germaine, ed. *Transforming Body Image*. Freedom, Calif.: Crossing Press, 1985.

Jaffe, Dennis T., Ph.D., and Cynthia D. Scott, Ph.D. *Self-Renewal*. New York: Simon & Schuster, 1989. (Originally published as *From Burnout to Balance*. New York: McGraw-Hill, 1984.)

Justice, Blair, Ph.D. *Who Gets Sick?* Houston: Peak Press, 1987.

Marx, Ina. *Fitness for the Unfit: The Way to a New Beginning*. New York: Citadel Press, 1990.

Matthews-Simonton, Stephanie, O. Carl Simonton, and James L. Creighton. *Getting Well Again*. New York: Bantam Books, 1976.

Miller, Emmett E., M.D. *Self-Imagery: Creating Your Own Good Health*. Berkeley: Celestial Arts, 1986.

Moyers, Bill. *Healing and the Mind*. New York: Bantam Doubleday Dell Publishing Group, 1993.

Ornish, Dean. *Dr. Dean Ornish's Program for Reversing Heart Disease*. New York: Random House, 1990.

Pitzele, Sefra Kobrin. *We Are Not Alone: Learning to Live with Chronic Illness*. New York: Workman Publishing, 1985.

Register, Cheri. *Living with Chronic Illness*. New York: The Free Press, 1987.

Ryan, Regina Sara, and John W. Travis. *Wellness: Small Changes You Can Use to Make a Big Difference*. Berkeley: Ten Speed Press, 1991.

Sanford, John A. *Healing and Wholeness*. New York: Paulist Press, 1977.

Schneider, Meir. *Self Healing: My Life and Vision*. London: Rutledge and Kegan Paul, 1987.

Selye, Hans, M.D. *The Stress of Life*. New York: McGraw-Hill, 1956; rev. ed., 1975.

Weil, Andrew, M.D. *Health and Healing: Understanding Conventional and Alternative Medicine*. Boston: Houghton Mifflin, 1983.

——. *Natural Health, Natural Medicine*. Boston: Houghton Mifflin, 1991.

Weiner, Florence. *No Apologies*. New York: St. Martin's Press, 1986.

CREATIVITY AND HUMAN POTENTIAL

Abrams, Jeremiah, ed. *Reclaiming the Inner Child*. Los Angeles: Jeremy P. Tarcher, 1990.

Bandler, Richard, and John Grinder. *Frogs into Princes*. Moab: Real People Press, 1979.

———. *Using Your Brain—for a CHANGE*. Moab: Real People Press, 1985.

Bradshaw, John. *Homecoming: Reclaiming and Championing Your Inner Child*. New York: Bantam Books, 1990.

Bry, Adelaide, and Marjorie Bair. *Directing the Movies of the Mind: Visualization for Health and Insight*. New York: Harper & Row, 1978.

Buzan, Tony. *Use Both Sides of Your Brain*. New York: E. P. Dutton, 1974, 1983.

Covey, Stephen R. *The 7 Habits of Highly Effective People*. New York: Simon & Schuster, 1989.

Davis, Bruce, Ph.D. *The Magical Child Within You*. Berkeley: Celestial Arts, 1982.

de Bono, Edward. *Lateral Thinking*. New York: Harper & Row, 1970.

De Laney, Gayle. *Living Your Dreams*. San Francisco: Harper & Row, 1988.

Ferguson, Marilyn. *The Aquarian Conspiracy: Personal and Social Transformation in the 1980's*. Los Angeles: Jeremy P. Tarcher, 1980.

Gawain, Shakti. *Creative Visualization*. New York: Bantam Books, 1978.

Goldberg, Philip. *The Intuitive Edge*. Los Angeles: Jeremy P. Tarcher, 1983.

Gregory, R. L. *The Intelligent Eye*. New York: McGraw-Hill, 1970.

Harman, Willis, and Howard Rheingold. *Higher Creativity: Liberating the Unconscious for Breakthrough Insights*. Los Angeles: Jeremy P. Tarcher, 1984.

Hillman, Anne. *The Dancing Animal Woman*. Norfolk, Conn.: Bramble Books, 1994.

Huxley, Aldous. *The Doors of Perception*. New York: Harper & Row, 1954.

Koberg, Don, and Jim Bagnell. *The Universal Traveler*. Los Altos: William Kaufman, 1973.

N.E. Thing Enterprises. *Magic Eye: A New Way of Looking at the World*. Kansas City: Andrews and McNeel, 1993.

———. *Magic Eye II: Now You See It*. Kansas City: Andrews and McNeel, 1994.

Noonan, Peggy. *Life, Liberty and the Pursuit of Happiness*. New York: Random House, 1994.

Pearce, Joseph C. *The Magical Child*. New York: Bantam Books, 1986.

Pelletier, Kenneth R. *Mind as Healer, Mind as Slayer*. New York: Dell, 1977.

Redfield, James. *The Celestine Prophecy: An Adventure*. New York: Warner Books, 1993.

Smothermon, Ron, M.D. *Winning Through Enlightenment*. San Francisco: Context Publications, 1980.

von Oech, Roger, Ph.D. *A Whack on the Side of the Head*. New York: Warner Books, 1983.

Waitley, Denis E., Ph.D. *Seeds of Greatness*. New York: Simon & Schuster, 1983.

Whitfield, Charles L., M.D. *Healing the Child Within*. Deerfield Beach, Fla.: Health Communications, 1987.

WOMEN, MEN, AND RELATIONSHIPS

Berne, Eric, M.D. *Games People Play*. New York: Ballantine Books, 1964.

Bettelheim, Bruno. *A Good Enough Parent*. New York: Alfred A. Knopf, 1987.

———. *The Uses of Enchantment: The Meaning and Importance of Fairy Tales*. New York: Random House, 1975.

Bly, Robert. *Selected Poems*. New York: Harper & Row, 1986.

Erikson, Erik H. *Childhood and Society*. New York: W. W. Norton, 1950.

———. *Insight and Responsibility*. New York: W. W. Norton, 1964.

Hendrix, Harville, Ph.D. *Getting the Love You Want: A Guide for Couples*. New York: Harper & Row, 1988.

John-Roger. *Relationships: The Art of Making Life Work*. Los Angeles: Mandeville Press, 1986.

Pearson, Carol S., Ph.D. *The Hero Within: Six Archetypes We Live By*. San Francisco: HarperCollins, 1989.

Welwood, John, Ph.D. *Journey of the Heart*. New York: HarperCollins, 1990.

Williamson, Marianne. *A Woman's Worth*. New York: Random House, 1993.

PSYCHOLOGY AND THE SPIRIT

Bennett, Hal Zina, Ph.D., and Susan J. Sparrow. *Follow Your Bliss: Let the Power of What You Love Guide You to Personal Fulfillment in Your Work and Relationships*. New York: Avon Books/Morrow, 1990.

Bennett, Hal Zina, Ph.D. *The Lens of Perception*, 2d ed. Berkeley, California: Celestial Arts, 1994.

Bennett, William J. *The Book of Virtues: A Treasury of Great Moral Stories*. New York: Simon & Schuster, 1993.

Borysenko, Joan, Ph.D. *Fire in the Soul: A New Psychology of Spiritual Optimism*. New York: Warner Books, 1993.

———. *Guilt is the Teacher, Love is the Lesson.* New York, Warner Books, 1990.

———. *Minding the Body, Mending the Mind.* Reading, Mass.: Addison-Wesley, 1987.

Bradshaw, John. *Healing the Shame that Binds You.* Deerfield Beach, Fla.: Health Communications, 1988.

Branden, Nathaniel. *Honoring the Self.* Los Angeles: Jeremy P. Tarcher, 1983.

———. *The Psychology of Self-Esteem.* New York: Bantam Books, 1969.

Campbell, Joseph, Ed. *The Portable Jung.* New York: Penguin Books, 1971.

Campbell, Joseph, with Bill Moyers. *The Power of Myth.* New York: Doubleday, 1988.

Coit, Lee. *Listening: How to Increase Awareness of Your Inner Guide.* Tiburon, Calif.: The Foundation for Inner Peace, 1985.

———. *Listening Still: How to Increase Your Acceptance of Perfection.* Tiburon, Calif.: The Foundation for Inner Peace, 1985.

Grof, Stanislav, M.D., with Hal Zina Bennett, Ph.D. *The Holotropic Mind: The Three Levels of Consciousness and How They Shape Our Lives.* San Francisco: HarperCollins, 1992.

Harman, Willis, Ph.D. *Global Mind Change.* Indianapolis: Knowledge Systems, 1988.

———. *Love Is Letting Go of Fear.* New York: Bantam Books, 1970.

Jampolsky, Gerald G., M.D. *Love Is the Answer.* New York: Bantam Books, 1991.

———. *Teach Only Love: The Seven Principles of Attitudinal Healing.* New York: Bantam Books, 1983.

Jampolsky, Gerald G. M.D. and Diane Cirincione. *Change Your Mind, Change Your Life.* New York: Bantam books, 1993.

———. *Wake-Up Calls.* Santa Monica: Hay House, 1992.

John-Roger and Peter McWilliams. *Do It!* Los Angeles: Prelude Press, 1991.

———. *Life 101.* Los Angeles: Prelude Press, 1990.

———. *You Can't Afford the Luxury of a Negative Thought.* Los Angeles: Prelude Press, 1988.

Jung, Carl G. *Man and His Symbols.* New York: Doubleday, 1964.

———. *Memories, Dreams and Reflections,* edited by Aniela Jaffe. New York: Random House, 1961.

Kabat-Zinn, Jon. *Wherever You Go, There You Are.* New York: Hyperion, 1994.

Kingma, Daphne Rose. *Random Acts of Kindness.* Emeryville, Calif.: Conari Press, 1993.

LeShan, Lawrence. *How to Meditate.* New York: Bantam Books, 1984.

Maslow, Abraham. *Toward a Psychology of Being*, 2nd ed. New York: Van Nostrand, Reinhold, 1968.

May, Rollo. *Love and Will*. New York: Delta Books, 1969.

Miller, Alice. *The Drama of the Gifted Child*. New York: Basic Books, 1981. (Original title: *Prisoners of Childhood*.)

———. *For Your Own Good*. New York: Farrar, Straus, Giroux, 1983.

———. *Pictures of Childhood*. New York: Farrar, Straus, Giroux, 1986.

Rogers, Carl L. *A Way of Being*. Boston: Houghton Mifflin, 1980.

Segal, Jeanne, Ph.D. *Living Beyond Fear*. North Hollywood, Calif.: New Castle Publishing, 1987.

Semigran, Candace. *One-Minute Self-Esteem: The Gift of Giving*. Santa Monica: Insight Publishing, 1988.

Siegel, Bernie S., M.D. *Love, Medicine & Miracles*. New York: Harper & Row, 1986.

———. *Peace, Love & Healing*. New York: Harper & Row, 1989.

Simon, Sidney B., Ed.D., and Suzanne Simon. *Forgiveness*. New York: Warner Books, 1990.

Sontag, Susan. *Illness as Metaphor*. New York: Farrar, Straus & Giroux, 1978.

Wilber, Ken. *Eye to Eye: The Quest for the New Paradigm*. Garden City, N.Y.: Anchor Press/Doubleday, 1983.

PASSAGE FROM LIFE INTO DEATH

Benjamin, Harold H., Ph.D. *From Victim to Victor*. Los Angeles: Jeremy P. Tarcher, 1987.

Cousins, Norman. *Anatomy of an Illness as Perceived by the Patient*. New York: W. W. Norton, 1979.

———. *Head First: The Biology of Hope*. New York: E. P. Dutton, 1989.

Deepak, Chopra, M.D. *Ageless Body, Timeless Mind: The Quantum Alternative to Growing Old*. New York: Random House, 1993.

Kubler-Ross, Elisabeth. *Working It Through*. New York: Macmillan, 1982.

LeShan, Lawrence. *Cancer as a Turning Point*. New York: E. P. Dutton, 1990.

Levine, Stephen. *A Gradual Awakening*. New York: Anchor Books, 1979.

———. *Healing into Life and Death*. Garden City, N.Y.: Anchor Press/Doubleday, 1987.

———. *Who Dies? An Investigation of Conscious Living and Conscious Dying*. New York: Anchor Books, 1989.

Moss, Richard, M.D. *How Shall I Live?* Berkeley: Celestial Arts, 1985.

Wilbur, Ken. *Grace and Grit*. Boston: Shambhala Publications, 1991.

THE SPIRITUAL JOURNEY

Andrews, Frank. *The Art and Practice of Loving.* Los Angeles: Jeremy P. Tarcher, 1991.

The Bible

Bly, Robert. *The Kabir Book: Forty-four of the Ecstatic Poems of Kabir.* Boston: Beacon Press, 1971.

Bolles, Richard N. *How to Find Your Mission in Life.* Berkeley: Ten Speed Press, 1991.

Cleland, Max. *Strong at the Broken Places.* Atlanta, Cherokee Publishing, 1986.

A Course in Miracles. Glen Ellen, Calif.: Foundation for Inner Peace, 1976.

Dass, Ram. *Be Here Now.* New York: Crown Publishing, 1971.

Dass, Ram, and Paul Gorman. *How Can I Help?* New York: Alfred A. Knopf, 1987.

Dossey, Larry, M.D. *Healing Words: The Power of Prayer and the Practice of Medicine.* New York: HarperCollins, 1993.

———. *Recovering the Soul.* New York: Bantam Books, 1989.

Feldman, Christian and Jack Kornfield. *Stories of the Spirit, Stories of the Heart: Parables of the Spiritual Path Around the World.* New York: HarperCollins, 1992.

Frankl, Viktor E. *Man's Search for Meaning.* New York: Simon & Schuster, 1959. (First published by Beacon Press, Boston, 1959.)

Fritz, Robert. *The Path of Least Resistance.* Salem, Mass.: Stillpoint Publishing, 1984.

Gallagher, Blace Marie. *Meditations with Teilhard de Chardin.* Santa Fe: Bear, 1988.

Gawain, Shakti. *Living in the Light.* Mill Valley, Calif.: Whatever Publishing, 1986.

Gibran, Kahlil. *The Prophet.* New York: Alfred A. Knopf, 1923.

Golas, Thaddeus. *The Lazy Man's Guide to Enlightenment.* New York: Bantam Books, 1980.

Goleman, Daniel. *The Meditative Mind: The Varieties of Meditative Experience.* Los Angeles: Jeremy P. Tarcher, 1988.

Hanh, Thich Nhat. *Being Peace.* Berkeley: Parallax Press, 1987.

———. *The Miracle of Mindfulness: A Manual of Meditation.* Boston: Beacon Press, 1976.

———. *Peace Is Every Step.* New York: Bantam Books, 1991.

———. *Touching Peace: Practicing the Art of Mindful Living.* Berkeley: Parallax Press, 1992.

Jampolsky, Gerald G., M.D. *Children as Teachers of Peace.* Berkeley: Celestial Arts, 1982.

————. *Out of Darkness into the Light: A Journey of Inner Healing*. New York: Bantam Books, 1989.

John-Roger. *The Way Out Book*. Los Angeles: Baraka Press, 1980.

————. and Peter McWilliams. *We Give to Love: Giving Is Such a Selfish Thing*. Los Angeles: Prelude Press, 1993.

Kavanaugh, Phillip, M.D. *Magnificent Addiction*. Lower Lake, Calif.: Aslan Publishers, 1992.

Millman, Day. *Way of the Peaceful Warrior*. Tiburon, Calif.: H. J. Kramer, 1980.

Peck, M. Scott, M.D. *The Road Less Traveled*. New York: Simon & Schuster, 1978.

Prather, Hugh. *Notes on Love and Courage*. New York: Doubleday, 1977.

Roekard, Karen G. R. *The Santa Cruz Haggadah*. Capitola, Calif.: The Hineni, Consciousness Press, 1991.

Saionji, Masami. *The Golden Key to Happiness*. New York: Society of Prayer for World Peace, 1990.

Teilhard de Chardin, Pierre. *The Phenomenon of Man*. New York: Harper Torch Books, 1961.

Wellwood, John, Ph.D. *Journey of the Heart*. New York: HarperCollins, 1990.

Zukav, Gary. *The Seat of the Soul*. New York: Simon & Schuster, 1993.

For Further Listening

Music awakens the heart and intensifies the awareness of spirit.
While it is true that each person's experience of music is unique,
the power, vibration, and passion of music is incredibly profound.
Music that vibrates the air vibrates *us* as well and creates tremendous joy, upliftment, and freedom. Music that carries such spiritual
inspiration and promise enables us to "vibrate" to the same glorious
level. During such experiences, we release ourselves from hurts and
judgments and enter into unconditional forgiveness. We can be
moved to tears and feel cleansed and healed by listening to music.
The following is a list of compositions that have affected me very

deeply. This list provides interested readers with the opportunity of exploring music that has the qualities of beauty, loving, devotion, and compassion that reflect the seven personal keys you deepened in *You Are Not Your Illness*. It is a blessing for me to share the music that I love with you.

(***)   I recommend these compositions highly. Allow the magic of the music to transport you.

CLASSICAL COMPOSITIONS

***   J. S. BACH
Well-Tempered Clavier, Books 1 and 2

***   J. S. BACH
Orchestral Suite no. 3 ("Air on a G String")

***   J. S. BACH
"Jesus, Joy of Man's Desiring," from Cantata 147
(This music is used twice to end each half of the cantata; Bach fully communicates joy of the spirit. Unsurpassed.)

***   BARBER
Violin Concerto
Adagio for Strings
(These first two movements of the Adagio for Strings contain some of the most moving and beautiful music ever written in the twentieth century.)

BEETHOVEN
Piano Concerto no. 5 ("Emperor") second (slow) movement
Symphony no. 7, slow introduction (depicting the vastness of divine power)
Symphony no. 5
Symphony no. 9, especially slow movement
String Quartet op. 74 ("Harp")

BRAHMS
A German Requiem
Symphony no. 1, slow movement

CHOPIN
Nocturnes
(Arthur Rubinstein, piano, RCA Red Seal)

COPLAND
Appalachian Spring (filled with passages containing a very tender, poetic inspiration)
Quiet City

DEBUSSY
Preludes for Piano, Book 1, no. 8 ("La Fille aux Chevaux de Lin")
La Mer

DVORAK
New World Symphony
(Leonard Bernstein, New York Philharmonic)

ELGAR
"Enigma" Variation no. 9 ("Nimrod")

*** HANDEL
Messiah
Concerti Grossi op. 3
Concerti Grossi op. 6

MAHLER
Symphony no. 2 ("Resurrection"): "O roschen Rot"

MOZART
Requiem
"Ave Verum Corpus" (well-known, heavenly choral piece)
Eine Kleine Nachtmusik

*** PACHELBEL
Canon in D
(Music is filled with compassion and love; I particularly like the version that is mixed with ocean sounds.)

*** SATIE
Piano Works
(Aldo Ciccolini, piano, EMI Classics)

*** RICHARD STRAUSS
Also Sprach Zarathustra
(Great opening, used in *2001: A Space Odyssey*, signifies our evolution into higher consciousness.)
Four Last Songs ("Abendrot")
(Captures the essence of letting go of earthly life and moving on to a higher level.)

*** RAVEL
Daphnis et Chloe Suite
(amazing opening)
"The Fairy Garden"
(Last movement of *Mother Goose Suite*, communicates a sense of
sweetness, love, and fulfillment, as in dreams coming true.)

VAUGHN WILLIAMS (A very mystical composer—communicates directly the essence of divine spiritual love through music, particularly in the following compositions.)

*** Symphony no. 5
(beautiful slow third movement and ending)
"Serenade to Music"
(Shakespeare's poetry set to music)
Symphony no. 6
"Lark Ascending"

*** WAGNER
Parsifal
(The prelude and ending of this opera are pure genius; based on
legend of the Holy Grail.)

INSPIRATIONAL/UPLIFTING
POPULAR MUSIC

A principle behind a lot of New Age music is to include a spiritually
uplifting quality. The following are some of my favorites.

*** Chant
The Benedictine Monks of Santo Domingo de Silos
Angel Records

Piano Sampler, volumes 1 and 2
Windham Hill Records

WILLIAM ACKERMAN
Conferring with the Moon
Windham Hill Records

PATRICK BALL
Celtic Harp: The Music of Turlough O'Carolan
Fortuna Records

PATRICK BALL
Celtic Harp, vol. II
Fortuna Records

TEJA BELL/STEVE KINDLER
Dolphin Smiles
Global Pacific Records

HAROLD BUDD/DANIEL ENO *with* DANIEL LANOIS
The Pearl
Caroline Records

BRUCE COCKBURN
Dancing in the Dragon's Jaws ,
Columbia Records

CHRISTOPHER COLUCCI
Wandering
The Force of Circumstance
Compositions for guitar and ensemble
Available from the artist:
6822 Ridge Avenue
Philadelphia, PA 19128

*** RUSTY CRUTCHER
Machu Picchu Impressions
Emerald Green Sound Productions

DEEP FOREST
Deep Forest
550 Music

BRIAN ENO
Ambient 1 Music for Airports
Caroline Records

ENYA
Watermark
*** *Shepherd Moons*
Reprise Records

JAMES GALWAY
Enchanted Forest
Vivaldi: The Four Seasons
RCA

PHILIP GLASS
Solo Piano
(All music composed and performed by artist.)
Columbia Records

AMY GRANT
The Collection
A & M Records

STEVEN HALPERN
Starborn Suite
Spectrum Suite
Sound Records (RX)

HIMEKAMI
Snow Goddess
Moon Water
Higher Octave Music

PAUL HORN
The Peace Album
Celestial Harmonies

KEITH JARRETT
Bridge of Light
ECM new series
*** *The Köln Concert*
Polygram Records

MICHAEL JONES
Pianoscapes
Michael's Music
Seascapes
Narada Productions

KITARO
Silk Road
Kitaro-Ki
Kojiki
Geffen Records

DANIEL KOBIALKA
Path of Joy
Timeless Motion
Fragrances of a Dream
Li-Sem Enterprises

DAVID LANZ
Return to the Heart
*** *Cristofori's Dream*
Narada Productions

DAVID LANZ/PAUL SPEER
Desert Vision
Natural States
Narada Productions

MANHEIM STEAMROLLER
The Christmas Collection, AGC 1984
Fresh Aire, volumes 1 through 4
American Gramophone

PATRICK O'HEARN
Ancient Dreams
Private Music

MIKE ROWLAND
The Fairy Ring
Music Design
And So to Dream
Arcade Music

IRA STEIN AND RUSSEL WALDER
Elements
Windham Hill

PAUL SIMON
Graceland
Warner Brothers

Songs My Children Taught Me
Windham Hill Records

Tri Atma
Higher Octave Music

TUCK AND PATTI
Love Warriors
Tears of Joy
Windham Hill Records

ANDREAS VOLLENWEIDER
Dancing with the Lion
*** *White Winds*
Caverna Magica
CBS Records

ROB WHITESIDES-WOO
Miracles

Sojourn (composed by Scott Fitzgerald)
From Heart to Crown
*** *Sacred Journey*
Search for Serenity Through a Course of Miracles
Search for Serenity Through Forgiveness
(Narrated by Leigh Taylor-Young)
Now Productions
P. O. Box 3925
Los Angeles, CA 90051

PAUL WINTER
Wintersong
Earthbeat
Living Music Records

YANNI
Reflections of Passion
Keys to Imagination
Private Music

MUSIC SOUND TRACKS FROM FILMS

MOZART
Amadeus
Fantasy Records

An Affair to Remember
Epic Records

ALEN MENKEN
Beauty and the Beast
Disney Records

VANGELIS
Blade Runner
Atlantic Records

JOHN RUTTER
Brother Sun, Sister Moon
American Gramaphone

VANGELIS
Themes
Chariots of Fire
Polygram Records

Cinema Paradiso
DRG Records

*** JOHN WILLIAMS
Close Encounters Sound Track
Z. Mehta, Los Angeles Philharmonic
Varese Sarabande

*** JOHN BARRY
Dances with Wolves
Epic

Dr. Zhivago
Sony Music

Field of Dreams
Nevus Records

MARK ISHAM
Film Music
Windham Hill

PATRICK DOYLE
Henry V
EMI Records

*** ENNIO MORRICONE
The Mission
Virgin Records

*** JOHN BARRY
Out of Africa
MCA Records

RICHARD ROBBINS
Room with a View
DRG Records

JOHN BARRY
Somewhere in Time
MCA Records

*** JOHN WILLIAMS
Star Wars Sound Track
Fox Records

MICHAEL NYMAN
The Piano
Virgin Records

*** MARK KNOPFLER
The Princess Bride
Warner Brothers

Resources

Because the pathway of choice to healing, recovery, or to a cure is an individual one, I have compiled a directory of resources. These resources have been helpful to me and to others who seek physical, mental, emotional, and spiritual support. They will also be of use to people who look beyond physical healing to an enhanced experience of personal wholeness.

Sources for information on treatment options, professional services and organizations, hot lines, learning centers, and regional agencies are listed in the pages that follow. Whatever choice you make, be authentic in expressing the deepest level of self-love possible.

I hope these resources will be of help to you and your loved ones. You are not alone anymore.

GOVERNMENT AGENCIES

ADA
Office on the Americans with Disabilities Act
Civil Rights Division
U.S. Department of Justice
P.O. Box 66118
Washington, DC 20035-6118
(202) 514-0301 (voice)

ADA HOT LINE
(800) 949-4232
(To reach your regional disability and business technical assistance centers.)

ADA NETWORK
(713) 520-0232

NATIONAL ORGANIZATION ON DISABILITY
910 Sixteenth Street, NW
Washington, DC 20006
(202) 293-5960; FX (202) 293-7999

ORGANIZATIONS

Aids Information Resources (or contact your local health department)

AMFAR
(800) 243-7909

NATIONAL AIDS INFORMATION CLEARINGHOUSE
(800) 458-5231

NATIONAL HIV/AIDS HOT LINE
Centers for Disease Control
(Questions and answers)
(800) 342-AIDS
(800) 394-7432 (Spanish)

Aids: Information Sourcebook, 1991–92

Oryx Press
4041 North Central Avenue at Indian School Road, Suite 700
Phoenix, AZ 85012-3397
(800) 279-ORYX; FX (602) 279-4663
Price: $39.95

Aids Treatment Information Services

AIDS LIBRARY OF PHILADELPHIA
32 North 3rd Street
Philadelphia, PA 19106
(215) 922-5120

AIDS LIBRARY OF SOUTH FLORIDA
175 NE 36th Street
Miami, FL 33137
(305) 537-6010

NEW YORK CITY AIDS LIBRARY
New York City Department of Health
(212) 788-4280

PROJECT INFORM
From San Francisco: (415) 558-9051
From California: (800) 334-7422
From all other states: (800) 822-7422

Aids Spiritual Support Services

Manhattan Center for Living (212) 533-3550
Los Angeles Center for Living (213) 850-0877
Friends in Deed (212) 925-2009

Cancer Information Resources

AMERICAN CANCER SOCIETY (ACS)
777 Third Avenue
New York, NY 10017
(800) 227-2345

AMERICAN CANCER SOCIETY
1599 Clifton Road, NE
Atlanta, GA 30329-4251
(404) 320-3333

THE AMERICAN SELF-HELP CLEARINGHOUSE
St. Clares–Riverside Medical Center
25 Pocono Road
Denville, NJ 07834
(201) 625-7101

THE CANCER FEDERATION
P. O. Box 52109
Riverside, CA 92517
(800) 982-3270

CANCER HOT LINE
(816) 932-8453

THE CENTER FOR ADVANCEMENT IN CANCER EDUCATION
300 E. Lancaster Avenue, Suite 100
Wynnewood, PA 19096
(610) 642-4810

COMMONWEAL
The Institute for the Study of Health and Illness
P. O. Box 316
Bolinas, CA 94924
(415) 868-2642

ECAP (Exceptional Cancer Patients)
1302 Chapel Street
New Haven, CT 06511

NATIONAL CANCER INSTITUTE (NCI)
Office of Cancer Communications
Building 31, Room 10A16
Bethesda, MD 20892
(800) 4-CANCER

NATIONAL COALITION FOR CANCER SURVIVORSHIP
1010 Wayne Avenue, Suite 300
Silver Spring, MD 20901
(301) 585-2626

NATIONAL HOSPICE ORGANIZATION
1901 N. Fort Myer Drive, Suite 901
Arlington, VA 22209
(703) 243-5900
(800) 658-8898

PLANETREE HEALTH RESOURCE CENTER
2040 Webster Street
San Francisco, CA 94115
(415) 923-3681

WELLNESS COMMUNITY
Main Office
Santa Monica, CA
(310) 453-2200

BREAST CANCER
INFORMATION RESOURCES

THE NATIONAL ALLIANCE OF BREAST CANCER
ORGANIZATIONS (NABCO)
9 E. 37th Street
10th Floor
New York, NY 10016
(To receive the 1994-1995 64-page Resource List, send $3.00 and a self-addressed stamped envelope.)

LINDA CREED BREAST CANCER FOUNDATION
Bodine Center Room 1-310
111 S. 11th Street
Philadelphia, PA 19107
(215) 955-4354

ORGANIZATIONS AND NATIONAL OFFICES

AMERICAN DIABETES ASSOCIATION
National Service Center
1160 Duke Street
P. O. Box 25757
Alexandria, VA 22314

AMERICAN HEART ASSOCIATION
National Office
7320 Greenville Avenue
Dallas, TX 75231

AMERICAN LUNG ASSOCIATION
1740 Broadway
New York, NY 10019

AMERICAN LUPUS SOCIETY
National Office
23751 Madison Street
Torrance, CA 90505

AMERICAN MEDICAL ASSOCIATION
535 North Dearborn Street
Chicago, IL 60610

AMERICAN OCCUPATIONAL THERAPY ASSOCIATION, INC.
1383 Piccard Drive
Rockville, MD 20850

AMERICAN PARKINSON DISEASE ASSOCIATION
116 John Street
New York, NY 10038

AMERICAN RED CROSS
150 Amsterdam Avenue
New York, NY 10023
(212) 787-1000

THE ASTHMA & ALLERGY FOUNDATION OF AMERICA
1125 Fifteenth Street NW, Suite 502
Washington, DC 20025
(202) 466-7643

THE AMYOTROPHIC LATERAL SCLEROSIS ASSOCIATION
185 Madison Avenue, Suite 1001
P. O. Box 2130
New York, NY 10016

ARTHRITIS FOUNDATION
National Office
1314 Spring Street, N.W.
Atlanta, GA 30309
(800) 283-7800

DYSAUTONOMIA FOUNDATION, INC.
370 Lexington Avenue
New York, NY 10017

EPILEPSY FOUNDATION OF AMERICA
4351 Garden Drive, Suite 406
Landover, MD 20785

THE JUVENILE DIABETES FOUNDATION
432 Park Avenue South
New York, NY 10016
(212) 889-7575

HANDICAPPED ORGANIZED WOMEN
P. O. Box 35481
Charlotte, NC 28235

LIBRARY OF CONGRESS
Division for the Blind and Physically Handicapped
Washington, DC 20542

THE LUPUS FOUNDATION OF AMERICA, INC.
National Office
P. O. Box 12897
St. Louis, MO 63141

MULTIPLE SCLEROSIS ASSOCIATION OF AMERICA (MSAA)
601 White Horse Pike
Oaklyn, NJ 08107
(800) 833-4672

MUSCULAR DYSTROPHY ASSOCIATION
National Office
810 Seventh Avenue
New York, NY 10019

THE NATIONAL MULTIPLE SCLEROSIS SOCIETY
733 Third Avenue
New York, NY 10017
(212) 986-3240

PARKINSON'S EDUCATIONAL PROGRAM
3900 Birch Street, no. 105
Newport Beach, CA 92660

SEX INFORMATION AND EDUCATION COUNCIL OF THE U.S.
(SIECUS)
80 Fifth Avenue, Suite 801-2
New York, NY 10011

UNICEF (United Nations Children's Fund)
3 UN Plaza
New York, NY 10017
(212) 326-7000

TOURETTE SYNDROME ASSOCIATION
41-02 Bell Boulevard
Bayside, NY 11361

UNITED SCLERODERMA FOUNDATION
P. O. Box 724
Watsonville, CA 95076

WORLD RESEARCH FOUNDATION
15300 Ventura Boulevard, Suite 405
Sherman Oaks, CA 91403
(818) 907-5483

GROUPS, ORGANIZATIONS, AND CLINICS

THE ACADEMY FOR GUIDED IMAGERY
P. O. Box 2070
Mill Valley, CA 94942
(800) 726-2070

AMERICAN CHRONIC PAIN ASSOCIATION
P. O. Box 850
Rocklin, CA 95677
(916) 632-0922

THE AMERICAN FOUNDATION OF TRADITIONAL CHINESE
MEDICINE
1280 Columbus Avenue, Suite 302
San Francisco, CA 94133
(415) 776-0502

AMERICAN HOLISTIC HEALTH ASSOCIATION
P. O. Box 17400
Anaheim, CA 92817
(714) 779-6152

AWARENESS AND RELAXATION TRAINING
Cabrillo College Stroke Center
501 Upper Park, Delaveaga Park
Santa Cruz, CA 95065
(408) 722-9005

CAMBRIDGE INSIGHT MEDITATION CENTER
331 Broadway
Cambridge, MA 02139
(617) 491-5070

THE CROHN'S DISEASE
COLITIS FOUNDATION OF AMERICA
444 Park Avenue South, 11th Floor
New York, NY 10016-7374

ECZEMA ASSOCIATION FOR SCIENCE AND EDUCATION
1221 Southwest Yamhill, Suite 303
Portland, OR 97205
(502) 228-4430

HERPES RESOURCE CENTER
P. O. Box 13827
Research Triangle Park, NC 27709
(919) 361-2120

INSIGHT MEDITATION SOCIETY
Pleasant Street
Bare, MA 01005
(508) 355-4378

INSIGHT MEDITATION WEST
P. O. Box 909
Woodacre, CA 94973
(415) 488-0164

THE INSTITUTE OF TRANSPERSONAL PSYCHOLOGY
744 San Antonio Road
Palo Alto, CA 94303
(415) 493-4330

INTERNATIONAL FOUNDATION FOR BOWEL DYSFUNCTION
P. O. Box 17864
Milwaukee, WI 53217
(414) 964-1799

SOCIETY FOR CLINICAL AND EXPERIMENTAL HYPNOSIS
128-A Kings Park Drive
Liverpool, NY 13090
(315) 652-7299

STRESS REDUCTION CLINIC
University of Massachusetts Medical Center
Worcester, MA 01655
(508) 856-1616

UNITED SCLERODERMA FOUNDATION
P. O. Box 399
Watsonville, CA 95077-0399
(404) 728-2202

PROFESSIONAL GROUPS

AMERICAN HOLISTIC MEDICAL ASSOCIATION
4101 Lake Boone Trail, Suite 201
Raleigh, NC 27607
(919) 787-5146

THE INSTITUTE FOR RELATIONSHIP THERAPY
1255 Fifth Avenue, Suite C-2
New York, NY 10029
(212) 410-7712; (800) 729-1121; FX (212) 410-7752

THE NATIONAL INSTITUTE FOR THE CLINICAL APPLICATION
OF BEHAVIORAL MEDICINE
Box 523
Mansfield Center, CT 06250
(203) 429-2238

THE SOCIETY OF BEHAVIORAL MEDICINE
103 South Adams Street
Rockville, MD 20850
(301) 251-2790

SERVICE ORGANIZATIONS

AMERICAN ASSOCIATION FOR MARRIAGE AND
FAMILY THERAPY
1100 Seventeenth Street NW, 10th Floor
Washington, DC 20036
(800) 374-2638

THE BIOFEEDBACK & PSYCHOPHYSIOLOGY CLINIC
The Menninger Clinic
P. O. Box 829
Topeka, KS 66601-0829
(913) 273-7500

THE HUNGER PROJECT (Global Office)
15 E. 26th Street
New York, NY 10010
(212) 532-4255; FX (212) 532-9785

INSTITUTE FOR INDIVIDUAL AND WORLD PEACE
2102 Wilshire Boulevard
Santa Monica, CA 90403
(301) 828-0535

KRIPALU YOGA FELLOWSHIP CENTER FOR YOGA AND HEALTH
P. O. Box 793
Lenox, MA 11240
(800) 967-3577; (413) 448-3400
(800) 546-1556

KUSHI INSTITUTE
P. O. Box 7
Becket, MA 01223
(413) 623-5741

MOVEMENT OF SPIRITUAL INNER AWARENESS (MSIA)
Box 3935
Los Angeles, CA 90051
(213) 737-4055

PEACE THEOLOGICAL SEMINARY & COLLEGE OF PHILOSOPHY
3500 West Adams Boulevard
Los Angeles, CA 90018
(213) 737-1534

SYDA FOUNDATION
Box 600
South Fallsburg, NY
(914) 434-2000

THE VERMONT TEDDY BEAR CO.
2031 Shelburne Road
Shelburne, VT 05482
(800) 829-BEAR

LEARNING CENTERS

ESALEN INSTITUTE
Big Sur, CA 93920
(408) 667-3000

FOUNDATION FOR INNER PEACE
(A Course in Miracles)
Attention: Robert Skutch, Director
Glen Ellen, CA 95442
(707) 939-0200

INSTITUTE OF NOETIC SCIENCES
P. O. Box 909, Department M
Sausalito, CA 94966-0909
(800) 383-1394

INTERFACE
55 Wheeler Street
Cambridge, MA 02138
(617) 876-4600

JOHN E. FETZER INSTITUTE
9292 West KL Avenue
Kalamazoo, MI 49007
(616) 375-2000

LANDMARK EDUCATION CORPORATION
(This organization empowers people to create new possibilities for living
life powerfully and effectively.)
353 Sacramento Street, Suite 200
San Francisco, CA 94111
(415) 981-8850

THE MIND-BODY MEDICAL INSTITUTE
185 Pilgrim Road
Boston, MA 02215
(617) 732-7000

NEW YORK OPEN CENTER
83 Spring Street
New York, NY 10012
(212) 219-2527

OASIS CENTER
7463 North Sheridan Road
Chicago, IL 60626
(312) 274-6777

OMEGA INSTITUTE FOR HOLISTIC STUDIES
260 Lake Drive
Rhinebeck, NY 12572
(914) 266-4301

PREVENTIVE MEDICINE RESEARCH INSTITUTE
900 Bridgeway, Suite 2
Sausalito, CA 94965
(415) 332-2525

RISE INSTITUTE
P. O. Box 2733
Petaluma, CA 94973
(707) 765-2758

THE SPIRITUAL EMERGENCE NETWORK (SEN)
5905 Soquel Drive, Suite 650
Soquel, CA 95073
(408) 464-8261

UNIVERSITY OF SANTA MONICA
2107 Wilshire Boulevard
Santa Monica, CA 90403
(310) 829-7402; FX (310) 453-5641

THE WORLD PEACE PRAYER SOCIETY
(The Peace Pole Project / The World Peace Prayer Ceremony)
800 Third Avenue, 37th Floor
New York, NY 10022
(212) 755-4755; FX (212) 935-1389

Acknowledgments

This book took a long time to write, and there are many people who generously helped me complete this work.

I am grateful for the teachings of Spirit that are woven throughout these pages. They have been manifested through my spiritual teacher, John-Roger, and find their way into my heart and into this work. I am forever grateful for his presence in my life.

I have been blessed with the rare opportunity to create with Hal Zina Bennett, Ph.D., my developmental editor and transcript consultant. A published author himself, Hal has been a loving angel of support to the book and to me as well. Because of his continual wisdom and guidance, combined with his gentle, perceptive criticism, I understood that finding my voice was, indeed, like climbing a mountain. And because of his unwavering commitment and insight, I was empowered to complete the upward climb to the top.

Elizabeth Frumin also did much to help bring the book to completion. She put in countless hours of creative and joyful support and proofreading, and offered suggestions for clarification that proved heartfelt and helpful. For their commitment, honesty and love, I am also deeply grateful to Joan Geller Solomon and Carol Guber for their unflinching emotional support, always reminding me that my word in the world is a reflection of my determination, my commitment to my purpose, and my unconditional devotion.

Heartfelt appreciation goes to Eunice Cordrey, for her extensive editorial support and technical assistance. Working with her has truly been a gift of the heart. Along with the encouragement of Michele Peters, Debbie Smith, and Judi Zwelling, this book has assumed its present form, outlasting two publishers, five editors, two title changes, and countless drafts of the manuscript. Many thanks to Ed Luoma and Al Willis at Reader's Forum, Wayne, PA., and to Christopher Colucci (Borders Books and Music Shop) and Erik Smith (Garland of Letters, Philadelphia), David Sand and David Stern (MSIA), Jeff Thomas (Sam Goody, Ardmore, PA), and Kellie Hansbrough and Bernie Kimble (WJJZ-101.6, Philadelphia) for helping me compile the discography.

Crucial to any creative work was the ongoing support of wayshowers, teachers, peers, and mentors. I have been blessed with the intelligence, wisdom, respect, and guidance of many gifted individuals on my path to mastership: John Morton, Jim Gordon, Barbara Shere, Ed Wagner, Roberta and Bertrand Babinet, Inez and Michael Hayes, Carl A. Ferreri, Gurudev (Armrit Desai), Barbara Knight-Meyers, Julio Kuperman, Werner Erhard, Cheryl and Paul Mychaluk, Mark and Sunny Shulkin, Ron and Mary Hulnick and Bernie S. Siegel all gently guided me back home—to the source of love, beauty, and grace that comes from within. From my heart, for the fellowship and loving we share in Spirit, I acknowledge all of you.

I was fortunate to connect with Toni Sciarra, my former editor from Prentice-Hall, who first caught the vision of this book and recognized its timeliness and importance. Thanks for your trust in me. To my editor, Becky Cabaza, for her excitement about the book's content: Thank you for your belief in me and your ongoing enthusiasm for this project. Your professionalism and creative judgment have made every aspect of this publishing process a joy to experience. To Bitite Vinklers and Diane Aronson for their commitment to copy editing with knowledge, intelligence and understanding. And for her steadfast empowerment, thanks to Marilyn Abraham, my editor-in-chief, and all the others at Simon & Schuster for not giving up on me a long, long time ago.

For my extended family of loyal friends and crystal souls: Audrey Reed, Zach Solomon, Gary Delfiner, Marilee Goldberg, Elizabeth Zeitlyn, Michele Benjamin, Barbara and Sylvan Cohen, Lou and Linda Tenaglia, Gail and David Torrence, Les and Lee Traband, Denis and Marylee Bischoff, Terry and Betty McCabe, Bob and Gloria Gable, Marlyn Kline, Elaine Radiss, Miriam Galper Cohen, Linda Liss, Marion Brodsky, Mario, Lucy, and Sabrina Morresi, John and Jothi Jurkofsky, David Epstein, Karen and Don Kaufman, Lee and Dani Nelson Noble, Marianne Sladzinski, Lesley, Karen, Shary and Gary Skoloff, Stevie Fisher, and to my spiritual family in the Movement of Spiritual Inner Awareness. You have guided me through the darkness and held me in my pain. My gratitude is deep and abiding.

Thanks also for the influence and support of Gary Green, Gloria Deva Brown, Larry Teacher, Al Lowman, Richard Petrino, Edna Tuttleman, Jillian Owen, Doreen Schwartz, and my physical therapists, Maria DiTullio, Gregory Biren, Felicia Greenfield, and Joanne Randall.

Heartfelt appreciation goes to Susan (Mashbitz) Smallow, Eve (Adelman) West, Frani (Steyer) Palman, Joyce (Arnold) Kear, Arlene Kaufman, Ellen (Pievsky) Gold, Elyce (Dubin) Redelheim, Joyce Becker, and Helene (Novzen) Aronberg. I have loved all of you for thirty-five years of rooted and enduring sisterhood and friendship.

Thanks to every person living a life of challenge who has supported himself/herself by attending my groups and lectures over the years. Your inspiration has given me continual courage and upliftment. You know who you are.

Hugs to my eighteen-year-old cats, Lucy and Sasha, for keeping me company, sprawling over my computer (even now!), and doing their *very* best to stay off my papers.

I am grateful to my brother, Stuart Noble, for his warmth, compassion, and belly laughter, and to the loving memory of my cousin,

Kenny Rossman. In your last days, you kissed my hand, held it to your cheek, and as we both felt the presence of angels, we found peace in the Light.

To the loving memory of Michael's mother, Muriel Topf. Her beauty and consistent encouragement throughout this endeavor kept me focused on the importance of this work.

To my parents for setting the example. There is so much to say that I must depend on your hearts to read between the lines. Your love and care have meant so much to me, as have all of life's passages we have moved through together: growing up, growing old, fighting and loving, hurts, illnesses, disappointments and healings, births, and deaths, and new life. For everything you've given to me, thank you for your patience, and Daddy, your determination has given me the gift of strength and hope. May God bless you both.

I want my readers to know that my husband, Michael, is at the very heart of this book. Michael has been so giving as an insightful and patient teacher, lover, magician, warrior, and the most supportive friend anyone could ever imagine as an unconditional partner on this journey of spiritual growth. Much of the courage and inner strength that are presented on the preceding pages, he has awakened within me. He is the one who yanked me away from a destructive "post-diagnosis" diet of chocolate, alcohol, cigarettes, depression, and negative thinking, and offered me an alternative lifestyle, to healthier living and inner healing: a possibility to triumph over resignation, of claiming my vulnerability as my strength, of hope, and of living my dreams. He is the one whose firm hands and fingers worked out the knots in my shoulders when I worked late hours. He is the one whose tireless encouragement guided me through the darkness, teaching me the true meaning of wisdom and surrendering to the way it is. He is the one who smoothed over my wounds with his music. He is the extraordinary one who made me laugh, bringing an ease and a gentle sweetness to my life that has lifted me beyond the sound and the light.

Thank you for your faith in me, for what we have learned together, and for making this all possible. I love you with all my heart.

And finally, thanks to the Divine Guidance that alone makes this and all works possible.

The Enduring One

The weak one fears to find her limits;
The foolish one oversteps his limits;
The strong one lives at the edge of her limits;
The wise one seeks to change his limits;
The enduring one has no limits;
For in the end, there is only God.

Reverend Michael Hayes